A story about waiting
My journey through paranoia hope and healing

A novel

QriquaS Mzolo

Contents

About the novel
- Chapter 1
- Chapter 2
- Chapter 3
- Chapter 4
- Chapter 5
- Chapter 6
- Chapter 7
- Chapter 8
- Chapter 9
- Chapter 10
- Chapter 11
- Chapter 12
- Chapter 13
- Chapter 14
- Chapter 15
- Chapter 16
- Chapter 17
- Chapter 18
- Chapter 19
- Chapter 20
- Chapter 21
- Postscript
- Endnotes

By the same author

First published in South Africa in 2021 by QriquaS Mzolo.

Copyright © Qriqua Sipho Mzolo

This is the work of fiction based on COVID-19. The characters and events are fictional, if an actual place it is used fictitiously any resemblance to real persons living or dead is not intended.

The right of QriquaS Mzolo to be identified as the author of A story about waiting has been asserted. No part of this publication may be reproduced, stored in a retrieval system, or transmitted in any form or by any means, electronic, mechanical, photocopying, recording or otherwise, without the written permission of the publisher.

Author's contact email qriquasmzolo@gmail.com

About the novel

The world was hit by coronavirus, an exceedingly small non-biological particle with only an outer membrane coat covering its genetic shell. When the pathogen enters the human cell, it creates a syndrome that complicates the functioning of the body to a point of death. Because of the rapid spread of the virus, the world health organisation declares it a pandemic of public health emergency and urges governments to do everything to shield citizens from its effects. The South African government declares a state of national disaster and promptly quarantines the country for thirty-one days. On the eve of a long-awaited trip to Amanzimtoti for reunion with his fiancé, the national shut down put the plans of a young doctor on hold for an indeterminate period. With four suitcases bundled in the boot of his old sedan-Honda Civic and no room to lay his head in, the doctor finds himself marooned. A brief conversation with his fiancé persuaded him crashing with a cousin in a commune at Kempton Park cannot harm him. Set against the backdrop of a small town east of Johannesburg, a town whose qualities– unrelenting and unquittable–many readers will recognise. The young doctor like the rest of the nation waits for the speedy lifting of the lockdown so things could get back to normalcy. Things take a sudden and unexpected turn prolonging his stay in Kempton Park. The promised relief: food parcels, financial grant, and the imminent arrival of vaccines gets pushed out then dashed. The broken promises aggravate the already grave situation precipitating an ugly turn of events no one could have predicted. Through the doctor's propulsive voice, the novel explores the experiences of the lockdown located in xenophobia, exclusion, lies and privilege. Given how disruptive the virus has been to every part of our lives I cannot imagine right now, but there will come a time when the pandemic is behind us. When that happens, then, it would be appropriate to ask, 'what the world would look like after COVID-19, if eligibility to work, socialize and travel were contingent on everyone holding an immunity passport? No story is perfect. The form does not permit perfection; it is too random, too complex, multi-layered, and too close to the messiness of life. A story about waiting is a journey through paranoia the collateral of madness.

Saturday, 25th March
Bae, I am on my way

For weeks now, I have tossed and turned in this bed with no television or radio to ease my insomniac sleep. At last, the day and the hour have come, I must live town tomorrow morning and come to you, my honey bunch, Ayobami. Everything is packed and the room I leave behind empty reminds me I should have already been there with you. I will not miss the friends I made here; I probably will not even remember the girl who asked me to become her husband a couple of weeks ago.

Do you remember the last night we spent together? The next morning, you woke up in a panic because you had slept through your alarm after our marathon of rolling in cotton sheets. You were running late for work and kissed me goodbye with your always almost too-wet lips on your way out. Then you stared at me deeply with that look someone gets when they were about to taste a juicy cheeseburger and said you would come visit soon. It was disarming. I believed it.

Remember when I said I appreciate transparency in a relationship? Well, I know spectres are supposedly see-through and all, but ghosting me is not exactly what I had in mind. And like all good ghosts, you have tried to haunt me. But I have got sage.

Do you remember how you said you have never felt so comfortable around someone after disentangling from my arms? That you felt like a nudist around me? How were you addicted to me? 'It is so easy being with you.' You said, and I laughed in disbelief. The stupid signature laughs your friends adore. And later that day, while walking through the park under the glaring sun, my arm held so tightly around your waist, I swear your legs could have fallen asleep at any moment. But you trusted I would carry you the rest of the way if they did.

I have said my farewells, wandered the familiar one last time, and watched ten-years of reality vanish like a steam. My heart yearns for what once was, despite the clarity of present jovialness. Not that I have become attached to this place. Sometime feelings of attachment are like that. However, there are unresolved fears related to attachment, knowing that one day everything changes. For once I jostled with my attachments to the place, I once called my own, to the version of myself I once loved, to the potentiality of a particular life that really would not be that bad once I have shaken all the depressing attachment.

Do not get me wrong, I am not afraid of moving on and forming new memories, familiarities, and intimacies. In fact, the feeling is urgent, restless, and relentless, murmuring the need to fly with my wings to be with you right now. Absence is efficacious. When I filled out my 2020 planner and bought my diary for the year, I forgot to leave empty spots to be filled later because I never imagined the year would turn out like this. 2020 may prove to a big unexpected surprise!

Although sleep stays away, last night I shut my eyes and pieces of the life I am leaving behind flashed in memory. I see the batik pillowcases in my bedroom your mom bought for my graduation. I see the bedside lamp you gave me for my 30th birthday. All of that is gone now what remains are the few things stuffed in the suitcase that I am taking with me.

Things that once gave me a sense of comfort are no longer the rejoinder to my story. I have donated lots of stuff to friends, few given to The Jerusalem Orphanage in Midrand. Two pieces of furniture a small table and stool given to Ntate Moabi, my neighbour who for the many years kept me entertained with Bassboy stories from his days as underground miner. A memory of his youth I suppose. I have taken the liberty to bring with me a single piece of furniture I recently bought from the auction, anticipating delivery by the courier there upon arrival. I hope you will like it.

This is it then. A chapter ending after years of hard medical study. I remember the early years of sweat and tears when the Departmental Head made me repeat modules that had nothing to do with medicine or pathology of sick bodies. I thought that was funny if not stupid. I remember taking odd jobs that filled my otherwise empty life. I leave no bad memories behind, however, the things that matter the most are inside me, locked up in my heart, a place of permanence that I will treasure forever.

Even for a seasoned driver like myself, the stretch to the coast can take its toll on the powers of concentration. I have done myself a favour enlisting the services of my friend as a co-traveller. I will wake up at dawn so I can avoid the highway traffic. Amanzimtoti the place you and I first met awaits to embrace me with love. Your love. I imagine a home right next to the sea with our names on it, with many rooms fitting for a family.

When I wake up in the morning, I will jump from this matrass reminding myself that it is for the last time I sleep on it. I will walk to the shower room, take no more time than is necessary and put on a track suite and be gone. Like wind never to be seen again. Never to return. I plan to grab a bite at the fast-food outlet along Shell Ultra City's filling stations on the N3.

It is early and quiet. The sky is still black. The world is asleep. In a few moments, the day will arrive roaring in its track. The stillness of dawn will be exchanged for the noise of the day, the calm and solitude will be replaced by the pounding pace of dailiness, the refuge of early morning invaded by decisions to be made. I am glad I made mine when there was still time a long time back. Doing life with you, Ayo.

Chichi has arrived, ready to trek the long haul. Leaning against the car hands inside his tracksuit pocket, he is not the talking type in the morning. I opened the car doors with the remote key lying next to the charger, I meet him outside we exchange pleasantries while I carry my suite cases into the boot and then climb into the front passenger seat.

Chichi opens the door and in one easy step got in. I drank in the familiar sight of him adjusting the mirror, settling in on the driver's seat adjusting height and distance for comfort relative to his height, shrugging forward to turn the key in the ignition. Then set up, draped his arms casually across the back of the seat as he looks almost disinterestedly over his shoulder ready to reverse the car. He stopped himself halfway through the manoeuvre as if immobilised by cramps in his lower abdomen.

He presses the button powering up the radio, which lands on 702 talkRADIO, my default station. At once we pick up a repeat announcement broadcasting government's declaration of the state of national disaster in terms of which we are asked to stay at home for 21-days starting midnight last night. I ask him if he knew about this, he nods his head saying he heard the news last night on eNCA channel. He had no way of reaching me because my mobile was off, and he apologises for his tardiness.

Naturally, I missed out on the breaking news. I have no TV in the room, my phone was off last night not wanting anyone to steal my earned peaceful sleep. While the car still idling, Chichi proceeded to update me that in terms of this announcement, we will not be permitted to travel across provinces without police permission, which permission will be a mission to obtain because police will insist that we give them several 'proofs' evidence of our emergency. 'It is better to delay the trip to a later time when things would have settled down.' His half counsel half admonishment sounds like anything but. I look at him with resignation in my eyes.

Sensing how distraught I am Chichi takes one look and says, 'I know how much you've been preparing for this day it must be disconcerting that on the last hour you are forced to postpone this trip. I am really sorry Bro. Tomorrow is yet another day, okay.' He put his arms around my neck and rubs his forehead against mine three times a bro code for solidarity. We keep quiet for a minute or so then he guides me to the boot of the car where we assist me to retrieve the four suitcases bundled there back to my room.

The room is bare, mattress the only piece of furniture standing against the wall its sparseness a reminder of what my life has become. Inside the room the echo is loud the sound is crude and grating. Sometimes I cannot hear myself breathing. I can hardly believe I must spend a day and another one after that and plenty more thereafter in this hole. But what choice do I have under the circumstances? Life has dealt me a bad hand.

Chichi leaves my room promising to return to check on me later in the day. I lay my head down for a moment while I collect my thoughts about what to do next, then fell asleep. I drift into half-sleep; my mind felt weighed down by an invincible mass.

Sometimes missing the sleeping world of unbounded adventure hurt my heart, it makes me long for you Ayo even more.

Thembisa is not the most glamorous neighbourhood one would write stories about and it tends to get a bad rap but there is nowhere else in the province where I could get a two-bedroom apartment with fully furnished kitchen for the rate I am paying. Where do I go to from here is a question I alone must resolve? I need do so speedily.

Something startled me with a fright I woke up for a second time. With the morning light sneaking through the sheet, I had made a curtain, had disturbed something that up till now I had succeeded in putting at the back of my mind. The light was grey, the sun's brightness tempered by the low-slung clouds. The air smelt of rubber and dirt and the soft smell of fallen rain.

It is ironic that I am advised to stay home to avoid death. For ten years my professional training prepared as well as conditioned me for nothing but to face death and its sting in the face, never to retreat from its ominous presence. Here I sit, finding myself taking and accept counsel from Chichi to tarry a little longer in Thembisa so I may avoid death. How sad.

Another bleak aspect of a pandemic we have all been forced to come to terms with is paying for our past actions. It can take a month for an uptick in infections to trickle down into hospitalisations and deaths. Baked in is how some choose to describe this grim arithmetic. Even when a lockdown has been imposed, for a time things only get worse.

Waiting is hard because it feels as if I am not doing anything, precisely the point of waiting–to do nothing - and that is difficult. Waiting transforms time into delay, and I bear delay with less equanimity if I think it avoidable. I try to wait patiently but most times not waiting at all. Waiting–patient, impatient, agitated and boredom–has many allotropes. Waiting for someone to finish the sentence, I want to shout, 'spit it out, you idiot,' and coerce the thoughtless, the sluggish, or merely incompetent, into speeding up. I resent being kept waiting even when the alternative is not attractive.

I have become a hermit entirely by accident, for fear others will suspect me of a thief. My lingering here may look like skulking, loitering, and then experience myself as an object of suspicion because I no longer have business to transact at the place where I have now become detained at. When you are alone, you lose your sense of who you are, because you do not have an image of yourself reflected in how other people react to you. I look at my watch repeatedly, signifying that I am up to neither good nor bad. This is a personal crisis and a time of reflecting. 'Is this what waiting does to a man?'

The country has been instructed that waiting at home to flatten the curve of the infection rate is care for self, for others, and for the hospital network. I do not know what is worse, the sacrifice demanded of me for the sake of shielding the vulnerable-the elderly-or enduring the strictures of the waiting game. I jot down a few notable observations to remind myself another day of this moment.

My mobile is ringing where it sits plugged. The screen fills with a photo of a brown-eyed shiksa goddess sticking her tongue sideways at the camera. I imagine her stretching on some seaside terrace, silk kimono pooling around her. My best friend is usually only awake at noon when she has been working the night before. I touch the icon and see that it is a message from Ayo responding to my earlier VN sent before I took a nap. I leap with joy.

Ayo regard my voice velvety. She insists I send her only voice notes instead of text or video messages, I on the other hand prefer that she sends me video notes I like the things she does with her face. I notice her scrunching up her small nose like she is just smelled something unsavoury.

'How thrilling,' she deadpans.'

'My neighbourhood is in full bloom. Beautiful. I had the anticipation that you would be walking in here at any minute now. And now this?'

'Listen hon, have the courage to accept what you cannot change, don't fight it. I will be here when the country opens cross-province travel whenever that will be. I miss you too. Lots.'

My Bae is mercurial and more than a little bit magical. It is not just me everywhere she goes people fall at her feet. She is the easiest to love and gives love freely and abundantly. She could make even quarantined lives feel expansive and lovely. But I also know she is fragile too. A membrane of skin stretches so thinly over her emotions it is always threatening to burst.

I do not know who is shaken the most. Her or me. But inside I know I am a miserable wretch, a guileless little man. In my thirties all I have managed to grow is a sense of self, akin to the transparent carapace of a soft-shelled crab. Heartbreak can pierce my thin hide and reduce me into smithereens. We weep when we must and rejoice when there is a reason to do so. She will never be silent when I am hurting. But for now, I must heed her advice to lodge with her cousins in Kempton Park.

Sunday, 26th March
The state of disaster

'Fellow South Africans, I am addressing you this evening on a matter of grave national importance. The world is facing a medical emergency far graver than what we have experienced in over a century. Given the scale and the speed at which the virus is spreading, it is now clear that no country is immune from the disease or will be spared its severe impact.'

'Never in the history of our democracy has our country been confronted with such a severe situation. This situation calls for an extraordinary response; there can be no half-measures. Cabinet held a special meeting earlier today, we have taken urgent and drastic measures to manage the disease, protect the people of our country and reduce the impact of the virus on our society and on our economy… accordingly, I announce that in terms of Section 12 of the National Disaster Act, cabinet has decided that a national lockdown effective from midnight Friday.'

…It is true that we are facing a grave emergency. But if we act together, if we act now, and if we act decisively, we will overcome it…It is these attributes of our national character [resilience and solidarity] that won us our democracy and it is what will ensure our victory over this pandemic…he exhorted the nation to be courageous, to be patient, and above all too show compassion. Let us never despair. For we are a nation at one, and we will surely prevail… If we work together, if we keep to the path, we know we must take, we will beat this disease. I have no doubt that we shall overcome.

…Much is being asked of you, far more than I should ever ask. But we know that this is a matter of survival, and we dare not fail. We shall recover. We shall overcome…. I have faith in the strength and resilience of ordinary South Africans, who have proven time and time again - throughout our history - that they can rise to the challenge. We shall recover. We shall overcome. We shall prosper… much has been asked of you, far more than should ever be asked. And we dare not fail. We shall recover. We shall overcome. I thank you.'

With those words, South Africa was quarantined. BOOM! On that day, the future forecasted pandemic arrived in one bang. On January 30th the WHO declared a global health emergency. 'We have therefore made the assessment that COVID-19 can be characterized as a pandemic.' The global health emergency was now officially a pandemic — the first one to be caused by a coronavirus.'

On the 5th of March is the day that marks the first reported and confirmed case of coronavirus in the suburb of Hilton, north of Durban. It would be 30 days later before we have our confirmed coronavirus related death in the country.

The president stood still for three maybe four seconds without even as much as betting an eyelid then, in a twinkling of an eye vanished leaving me transfixed to a vacant podium as though he was about to return to continue the address. I remember seeing my television screen changing into white, purple and lime revealing the OUTsurance advert over the by-line, 'You are never alone.'

The president had appeared measured and considered in his address to the nation. I could not say the same about his junior ministers who came across as brash, blustery, bombastic, and self-serving buffoons in moments when they should have shown compassion and maturity of leadership. A state of national disaster would be extended to what looked like in perpetuity. Gradually easing off the rules in terms of a Risk-Adjusted Phased approached – whatever that jargon means.

It was Barack Obama who said, 'the moral test of government is how it treats those who are in the dawn of life, the children; those who are in the twilight of life, the elderly and those who are in the shadows of life, the sick, the needy and handicapped.' This statement is self-evident not just as an ideal but as a north star that I live by and by which I am going to measure the moral worth of my government lead by its president. Fear is not a reason to decide who gets to live one way, who gets to live another. Surviving is not the goal, thriving and flourish is. We will not come through the coronavirus pandemic successfully unless everyone does.

Days running to the national lockdown, the nation had been glued on their television sets intently watching with horror a convulsing Wuhan Province under the weight of a viral assault. The Chinese infections were surpassed only by Italy, Spain, USA, UK, Brazil and India in terms of the number of deaths and the speed with which the infections happened. The drama that played publicly was concentrated. Weeks rather than months revealed the full horror of it. I realised at that time most of the world was scrolling, cast adrift in a sea of uncertainty, the news only a rising count of numbers of people dying from an unseen enemy.

The president ordered soldiers to keep vigilant watch over a frightened nation. For weeks, South Africa prepared for the arrival of the 'great storm,' with increasing fear and trepidation hours turned into days, days into months and eternity. As the anxiety increased the jittery nation looked to someone, anyone who would be bold to stand up and offer solace and encouragement to a nation in its darkest hour. None emerged. And so, by default the president became that figure, but was ill-suited. In each televised appearance the president appeared more nervous less assured than the previous appearance. People read his body language and somehow knew they were between the rock and the hard place. Fucked. Totally.

China had locked down the city of Wuhan on the 23rd January. Shortly after that, over two thirds of the world's population had at one time or another shut its borders down, ordered its people to shut their doors and lock themselves inside proof that we are inescapably part of a world in which microbes and the animals that transmit them don't know geographic borders.

On 11 March, the World Health Organization announced the COVID-19 virus to be a pandemic. From that moment, everyday life began to change. Firstly, restrictions between nations were introduced to protect people from passing infection around. Secondly, fear grew among the people, places, once full of life, were empty; interpersonal relationships changed. It was inevitable that South Africa was going to follow the advice of the WHO.

Shortly after 8 pm the government ordered the country to shut down, for communities to lock themselves indoors and follow the stay-at-home orders issued by the president. By that order, the country came to a standstill. The tide turned. Commuting stopped. Towns emptied. Pavement stalls cleared instantaneously as were construction sites, retail, and manufacturing factories. Workplaces grinded to a halt as were schools, universities, and churches. The taverns and beer halls lost their regular patrons. Shopping malls were the only sights where life was seen.

A one-metre-distance between persons in public spaces was regulated. Coughing or sneezing on to the elbow or with a disposable handkerchief was ordered, covering the mouth and nose became obligatory, so was the sanitising of hands and washing of hands for twenty seconds. Avoiding contact with crowds, and regular disinfection of public transport such as taxis was done. Orders are one thing, following them an entirely different matter. As in the scheme of things, none thought the rules were for their good they followed them only where policed compliance was evident.

Leading up to this announcement, government had recruited an eminent group of 51 top rated, world-renown scientists that included Epidemiologist, Virologists, Biostatisticians, top Physicians and Mathematical Data Modellers. This group was assembled by the Minister of Health to advise the cabinet and the president on how to respond to the spread of the virus, the most effective way of preventing infection and how to defend society from its deadly effects.

The Ministerial Advisory Committee an equivalent of SAGE in the UK was led by Professor Salim Abdool Karim, it fed information into the National Coronavirus Command Council that met frequently at Manhlambandlovhu. In the beginning stages of the life of this committee consensus was reached according to evidence-based science regarding the cause and effect as well as the best course of action that the government decision-making machinery would be based to manage the pandemic.

Halfway through its life, however, ministers usurped its power and appropriated its brilliance for themselves, with time the political command consulted the committee of experts less and less, in many instances selected the advice it proffered on political expediency grounds. Disagreements between the committee and the Minister of Health became unavoidable, the crater opened wide. Public splats became staple menu for the press, evidence of it falling apart obvious.

A senior government official privy to the decision-making process said that the president was informed 'by the best brains in the country' before he makes decisions, and that the lockdown was based on scientific evidence put before him and his bureaucrats. Hindsight is the best educator it became pitifully plain the president was hiding his own vulnerability in the face of the onslaught of an unrelenting enemy.

None of us had encountered this virus before. We had no immunity, no monoclonal bodies, no vaccine, and no treatment. This meant we were all at risk of catching the virus. We did not decide who caught the coronavirus that caused COVID-19 disease. We could not even try keep disease from spreading or seek measures to alleviate its effects on us or others. The decision to be sick or not was not given to us. We are at the mercy of the virus. Totally.

It was outside our control when the disease passed from one person to the next asymptomatically before anyone could protect us. It became a case of everyone for himself and God for us all. Paralysis was immediate. For as long as the threat remained, fear dwelt the hearts of the people. We were scared witless me included. For their part South Africans agreed with their president for once, that a hard lockdown followed by stay-at-home was necessary to prevent the virus wiping off the nation.

In his address to the nation the president spoke to two different audiences, which received his message variably. The first group of people consisted of the adults - grandpas, grandmas, moms, and dads. This group regarded president's instruction pertinent to their welfare and thought themselves fortunate to so instructed. They have seen death before and could smell it just a distance away creeping slowly by the doorstep ready to announce itself any moment. They took the president at his word. Literally. They cooperated with the authorities fully.

Makhathide an elderly neighbour told me she regarded the president's instruction as direct speaking of God. Makhathide never ceased to pray for the president and wished him and his family a long life. Shaping Makhathide's attitude and others like her was the loathsome thought of perishing alone at a government hospital like Thembisa, Livingstone, Dora Nginza or Mamelodi where none of their children would be allowed to wait by her side in her final minutes. Her bones would not be buried in a dignified manner in keeping with her fore father's tradition. Makhathide feared if death took her, her children would be dependent on an uncaring state she had witnessed in her living years. This thought had increased her restlessness and deepened her anxiety.

The second group that also watched the president's address arose to offer a different response. The young more naïve audience scoffed at the insinuation they were going to die because of the virus. 'Ai, uyahlanya uCup Cake, angek' isbambe ikhodvad. Eintlik thina vele as'fly, sibloma la emakasi wethu waya waya. Ayinajive nathi ikhovivi, siyizinja ze game.' Gung ho and defiantly dismissive, the level five total shut down announced by the president was promptly downgraded to level one disregarded any social protocols accompanying the instructions. Life continued like there was no nothing. The young people were hundred percent ignorant and hundred percent lucky at the same time.

Shops, malls, and other cool hangout joints were out of reach for this group. Between, 9am and 6pm streets were full of teens milling around apparently bored out of their minds, not knowing what to do with their empty lives questioning the pointlessness of it all. I would see them occasionally pulling back to hide behind stucco walls when a Saps patrol squad veered into the street to disperse accumulating mobs. They would gather again as soon as the patrol car vanished out of sight. One thing the coronavirus pathogen love is a gathered crowd.

Sunday, 28th March
My shadow haunts me

The sky turns bronze on the horizon, air a chilling bite as the sun sets. The beginning of lockdown marked the point of rupture with my former way of life. Overnight, people drained from the streets of our towns and cities as they disappeared into their homes. When the world stopped yesterday, many looked out the window. Absence became the hallmark of COVID-19. In our absence, nature found an opportunity. Birdsong boomed out over once busy highways and goats munched the roadside verges. Birdsong replacing car horns and brake scritches. Watching green buds emerge from the thawing ground. For those lucky not to have family fall ill, the passing flash of an ambulance siren along an empty street was sometimes all that suggested the growing death toll and crisis. In a moment of darkness, it was a wonderful balm to turn to nature. Hope giving.

I am sitting by the corner on a lone matrass emblematic of what the world has become, wearing a boxer short and robe trying to figure out what on God's earth has just happened and what am I supposed to do with the emptiness that surrounds me. I have no room to lay my head; I have given away all my belongings or what was left of it. I believe in living by the numbers. Twenty-five. This is the number I count to every morning before I open my eyes. It is a meditative technique to help my brain with memory, focus and attention, but the real reason I do this is because that is how long I take out of bed and to think about what I am going to do this day and the one after that.

Thirty-six. That is how many minutes I take to brush my teeth, take a shower, put on moisturiser and clothes for the day. Twenty-four. That is how many months I believe I should be dating a woman before she moves in with me. Thirty. The right age to get married. It is fifteen degrees outside; I know this because my ever so dependable smart phone constantly displays the readings. Practically a balmy winter weather by Gauteng standards which makes walking and jogging a breeze. Exercise outside is not allowed. Day one I am already falling apart. Great.

I force myself to look through the window in what was the kitchen nook overlooking Sereti street. I can see my reflection in the window. My figure appears somewhat larger than usual, as figures tend to be, and shows me older and in awful shape than I have ever been. Straight, shoulders back, my lips curved into a firm but benevolent smile. By moving my body backwards and forwards, more reflections of my visage appeared vexed and haunting.

I fix my gaze on the steadily building thin cirrocumulus clouds, then quickly morphing into cirrostratus formation in the firmament. My head tells me to go out contrary to the official instructions. Conflicted.

Tuesday, 29th March
We live in a sick world

While it may not be normal for my generation to experience a COVID-19 pandemic, it is common that disasters sweep through the world from time to time and from one generation to the next. This world is cursed with plagues, epidemics, earthquakes, heat waves, fire, hurricanes, tsunamis, famines, draughts, storms, snow floods, sickness, and death.

For example, we know as far back as Noahtic period floods wiped out humans and animals off the face of the earth saving only Noah and his family and a handful of beasts. In medieval antiquity, epidemics wiped out several millions of lives. One of the earliest known was the Babylon flu epidemic around 1200 BC. The Antonine Plaque between 165-180 had killed 5 million people. The plague of Athens in 429 BC killed close to 100,000 people.

The Plague of Justinian 541-542 killed between 30-50 million. Between the years 735-737, Japanese Smallpox killed 30 million more. SARS-CoV-2 the original not the variant appeared in Wuhan, China, in the sixth century. Black Death took place between 1347-1351 ending 200 million lives over 60% of European population. Smallpox that erupted during the 1520s ended 56 million lives.

The English Sweating sickness outbreak mainly in England during the summers of 1485,1508,1517,1528 through to 1551. This disease gained infamy because it killed its victims withing 24 hours of sweating to death. Death came swiftly after profound weakness and agonising shortness of breath culminating with chest pain, rapid pulse, and cardiac palpitations. Then the Sweating sickness disease vanished without a vaccine.

There were the 17th century plagues during the years between 1600 and 1700. The Cholera outbreak in 1817-1923 decimating some populations around 1million. The Third Plague in 1855 took away 12 million people. Yellow Fever was less deadly in comparison with other pandemics affecting only 100-150 thousand lives.

In 1901 in Cape Town, a plague epidemic produced an overly aggressive racial segregated quarantine that became the blueprint for future segregated towns and communities in apartheid South Africa. It is a stark example of how human bigotry often drives oppressive responses against those most marginalized in a society.

HIV/Aids around 1981-2020 took away an estimate of 35 million lives. Recently, we have seen infectious diseases like the H7N9 Asian flu, H1N1 Swine flu, Ebola, Lassa fever, West Nile fever, Zika, MERS, SARS and now the novel coronavirus breakout. We know how communities reacted in the aftermath of each outbreak. However, despite the phenomenal advances in medicine, most infectious diseases remain without a vaccine apart from Smallpox disease, which has since been eradicated.

Seventy five percent of the newly emerging diseases currently affecting humans originate in animals. Over the past 17 years there have been three major outbreaks of highly pathogenic coronaviruses: SARS-CoV in 2003, MERS coronavirus in 2012 and now SARS-CoV-2. Based on this history of having a highly pathogenic coronavirus emerge approximately every decade, we should expect to have to deal with more of the viruses in the near term.

While the general knowledge of the various viruses has been extant since 1192, it was not until there were advances in technology that the scientific community developed an appreciation of the pathogens. In 1931, Virologists were able to see the shape and size of the pathogens studied under a powerful electron microscope.

Coronaviruses were first identified around the 1960s. From then on, we knew that almost everyone gets a coronavirus infection at least once in their life, most likely as a young child. Epidemiologists have largely concluded that COVID-19 will likely become endemic because that is the nature of diseases. Take the Spanish Flu. Its first outbreak was the H1N1 flu, against which people had no defence. After a certain amount of time the H1N1 virus mutated into a less dangerous type, as a result the H1N1 became endemic. Every year a few of the people who have the flu have an H1N1 flu, as this subtype of flu viruses continue circulating at low levels, with mostly less aggressive strains. Occasionally, a more aggressive strain as in 2009 with the Swine Flu, but by now our bodies have developed higher defences against it.

The outcomes of all pandemics can only be two: either the disease is so aggressive that it burns itself out, as it probably happened with the sweating sickness, or it slowly becomes endemic, like it happened with the first plague, which lasted almost 300 years and the second like it lasted for 500 years which ended in 1960. In approximately 1855 the third plague pandemic started. This has been by far the least aggressive of the three known plague pandemics and is short because we anticipate by end of 2022 70% of the world population would have been inoculated providing enough herd immunity at global level.

After the initial outbreak, regular outbreaks continued for several decades (for instance, in 1900 localized outbreaks were recorded in Glasgow, San Francisco, Manila, Australia, and Russia, in 1912 the outbreaks had spread to Puerto Rico and Cuba). By the mid-century, though, the outbreaks had decreased in frequency and magnitude to the point where the WHO declared the pandemic closed, but plague remains endemic in many parts of the world.

Covid-19 is a very infectious disease that causes a moderate mortality around 2% higher than the seasonal flu, but lower than the plague. It is unlikely to burn out. We have the vaccines that will end the pandemic in a couple of years. But the disease will not disappear. The vaccines will make us resistant enough to prevent large scale outbreaks. We will still have a scattering of mild cases, and occasional local outbreaks although easy to control but cannot be eradicated.

Snowden, author of *Epidemics and Society: From the Black Death to the Present*, has predicted worse pandemics in the near term that will afflict this and the next generation. He has conducted a wide-ranging study that makes the connection between epidemic diseases and societal change. People in 1918 felt guilty and disloyal somehow if they got sick with influenza, so they lied about it and how people died. There are number of things we can we learn from the history without repeating the same old mistakes.

Pandemics are happening far more frequent in this century than before we do not know why this is so. We know for example of dengue fever, yellow fever, typhus, dysentery, malaria, tuberculosis, and typhoid disease. We know that societies reacted to those outbreaks in a way that reshaped social relations in their milieu.

Snowden's book is a comparative investigation of the medical and social history of the major epidemics, this volume touches on themes such as the evolution of medical therapy, plague literature, poverty, the environment, and mass hysteria. In addition to providing historical perspective on diseases such as smallpox, cholera, and tuberculosis, Snowden examines the fallout from recent epidemics such as HIV/Aids, SARS, and Ebola and the question of the world's preparedness for the next generation of diseases.

This sweeping exploration of the impact of epidemic diseases looks at how mass infectious outbreaks have shaped society, from the Black Death to today. Snowden reveals the ways that diseases have not only influenced medical science and public health, but also transformed the arts, religion, intellectual history, and warfare.

Epidemics are not random events that afflict societies capriciously without warning. On the contrary, every society produces its own vulnerabilities. To study them is to understand that society's structure and its standard of living and its political priorities. Epidemic diseases, in that sense have always been signifiers and the challenge of medicine is to decipher the meaning embedded in them.

Snowden says epidemics are living social laboratories. The effects of pandemics have changed how societies function and reshape social relations. They involve many actors not least of which is the microbe in question. Different microbes do affect people in different ways. Different people behave differently before an epidemic than during an epidemic and in the middle when they are tired of it.

Under certain circumstances, the passage of the diseases through communities has triggered large-scale and revealing responses among the members of communities at risk. These responses include stigmatization, scapegoating, flight and mass hysteria and riots. This was certainly true with coronavirus in certain parts of the world. Such events provide important lens through which to examine such affected communities – the relations of human beings to one another and the moral priorities of political leaders and the severely compromised living standards of the poor communities that were ignored in more settled times.

Hornby author of *Miss Austen* accounts for how fear of contagion informed the manners and mores of the English Regency many years back. In 1775, there was an outbreak of smallpox in Newbury, Berkshire. At that time, the disease was a regular visitor, bringing with its chaos and misery, and was always met with the most stringent measures.

In the rectory at Enborne, a few miles outside the town, the Lloyd family did what they always did to protect themselves: they went into what we now call lockdown. Nobody went out, and no-one but the most trusted servants gained entry. Still, the disease found its way in. The coachman, no doubt fearful of losing his position, concealed the fact that the virus was in his cottage. Smallpox ripped through all nine members of the Lloyd household.

Two of the adolescent daughters, Martha, who grew up to be Jane Austen's best friend, and Mary, who was to become Mrs James Austin, were both dangerously ill and bore the horrible scars for the rest of their lives. Their little brother, Charles, just seven years old, the treasured only son–did not survive. As was the custom, his doting parents were plunged into mourning. Though they stopped wearing black eventually, they never got over it. The coachman, no doubt fearful of losing his position, concealed the fact that the virus was in his cottage.

The effects of COVID-19 have put a break on social development. We have done a U-turn, travelled back, and our behaviour and concerns are suddenly so much more like those of the Regency period. After all, they lived by the rules of social distancing. They bowed, they curtsied. Yes, a hand might be kissed but, ideally, it was through a glove.

They crushed into ballrooms, certainly, and danced away the night, but there was none of that waltzing nonsense; pressing against the body of a stranger was for later, more relaxed times. They pirouetted around one another, walked side by side, approached and withdrew. And no intimacy took place until after the altar, when you were stuck sharing infections for good. Their lives were domestically centred.

Children were generally taught at home by a parent or relative. Unmarried adult offspring lived with their parents. Generations gathered beneath one roof, and the primary focus of everyone's concern was caring for, and respecting, the needs of the oldest among them. When Jane Austen's letters were first published, they were met with derision. This was all the greatest woman of the age had to say for herself.

Where were her thoughts on the war with the French or political reform? All she can talk about is her health and the weather and the garden and the neighbours and the food. Well, if you don't count our own rantings about certain members of the government, none of which, I suggest, will bear reading about in a few hundred years, what do we now have to say for ourselves? It's all pretty much about our health 'no symptoms yet, thanks.

But did you hear about so-and-so down the road? The garden, the new obsession of everyone lucky enough to have one. The weather: 'Thank God for the sunshine.' Now we see what it must have been like, when the elements turned against you and prevented your moment of statutory exercise. If we are doing this all again in November, we will be reduced to 'taking a turnabout across the room' like Miss Bingley and Lizzie in Pride and Prejudice.

So fine, then, if you happen to be in one of the larger stately homes. And, yes, the food. Sourcing it, cooking it, saucing it, and eating it have become the essence of our days. Down our way, barely a sentence is uttered that does not include the words 'supper' or 'lunch.' Austen herself wrote to her sister Cassandra of the impossibility of composing with her head full of doses of rhubarb and joints of mutton. The new 21st century worker from home will know just how she felt.

Researching the Regency by day, I then read contemporary novels by night. And there, I am back in that foreign country. They snog, they go to the pictures, they jostle in crowds. They imagine this have sex with people from other households. Woah! What? This is the work of a crazy person. Do none of these characters know they could catch something? Historical fiction seems so much more relevant these days. They lived with the ever-present fear of contagion, which ranged the country unchecked. And, for the first time in our lives, we are in their shoes.

A relative of Jane Austen's lost all three infant daughters to scarlet fever in the space of one week. The little girls' gravestone still stands in the churchyard at Steveston, arresting the hearts of all who stand there and read it. But have we ever before really understood what bereavement was like for them then? So many people lost children to sickness, wives and mothers in childbirth, whole swathes of their families to cholera, fevers, and tuberculosis.

It was different for them, though, wasn't it? All so common. Odds were against them. They knew to expect it. They did not need counselling or leave from work or any of that stuff. They just had to get on with it. And now we know. As our own death toll mounts and the numbers become so huge as to be almost incomprehensible, finally we know that short odds bring no sort of comfort.

The reverberations of a shift would be deeply felt. The entire field of redaction criticism of pandemic studies is dependent on nothing we know before now. If learning from previous outbreaks were to be our yardstick or sufficiently established, then redaction criticism will have to throw out everything from the last fifty years and start over again.

That baffling statistics are made up of terrible, individual tragedies. And perhaps soon, we might even bring back the custom of dressing in mourning. Then, as we grope our way back into normal life, we will see at once who emerges scathed, check our behaviour, and reach out in sympathy. Because we know that, like little Charles Lloyd's devastated parents, they might go on, but they will never get over it.

Like COVID-19, zoonotic diseases are becoming riskier to humans because of our own reckless actions. Our effect on the climate, encroachment on wildlife habitats and global travel have helped circulate animal-borne diseases. Combined with urbanisation, overpopulation, and global trade, we have set up an ideal scenario where we are in the season of more pandemics. Nipah virus is one of the WHO's top 10 diseases they believe is poised to be the next pandemic. Nipah has no vaccine, it is deadly, and there have already been a number of outbreaks in Asia recently.

Through the 6,000 plus years history of humanity there have been many bad years but never one that met every criteria Christ used to describe the run-up to his return. Some of these conditions have never all been so visible and simultaneously apparent. Nation shall rise against nation, and kingdom against kingdom: And great earthquakes shall be all over the place, famines and pestilences...' He explains that 'all these are the beginning of sorrows to come.'

God would have to show us pestilences in a new and visible way for this foretold condition to get our attention. He did with COVID-19, a global pandemic the world has seen nothing like since the 1665 Bubonic Plague. Yes, there have been pandemics in the past, and some more deadly but never in a world so fearful and interconnected as coronavirus. That we are in the middle of a prophesied condition is abundant. That this is the message God is sending us unmistakable. What that message might be is not clear.

Today's problems were foretold more than 2000 years ago, God knew this period would arrive and permitted it in its time. As the end of the age begins its final descent, the increasing troubles of this world impact us progressively. Harder times are coming our way before Jesus finally returns to end all suffering.

In Luke's account Christ added even more specifics. 'But take heed to yourselves, lest your hearts be weighed down with carousing, drunkenness and cares of this life and that day come on you unexpectedly. Watch therefore and pray always that you may be counted worthy to escape all those things that will come to pass and to stand before the Son of man.'

There is a difference between watching and being ready. Those who were ready went in with him – the bridegroom to the wedding. As the foolish virgins clamoured to be let in, they must have been shocked to hear the bridegroom answer, 'I do not know you.' People are invariably caught off guard and shocked by the suddenness of unfolding events, even when they have been warned. Being ready does not depend on what we know about the next coming pandemic but has to do with our spiritual condition. Anyone can see what is happening, but few can see where world events are leading.

It is considering the above, the most common command found in the Bible stands out to *not be afraid*. It is repeated 365 times. It certainly bears repeating. God never promised a crisis free life rather, he promised a way through the crisis. Jesus said, 'you will find trouble wherever you go. But take heart, I have overcome the world.' God is telling us to cast our anxieties upon him, the idea here being one of transference. To cast our anxiety, worry, and fear upon the Lord means that we transfer all of this to the Lord. When we do this, the anxiety is no longer ours because we have handed it to the Lord, so that it becomes his. The basis for this outsourcing is because the Lord he not only cares but has the arms to carry us. His yoke is light, and his burden is easy because he carries the burdens for us.

On this understanding, we can live carefree. On one level, we still care about the coronavirus, but on a higher level, it no longer bothers us because God takes care of it. For this reason, we appear to not care consequently, there's great liberty and freedom in the expression of our faith. People cannot be afraid when they know God is with them, and if he is with them, nobody can be against them.

Something in our nature finds it hard to heed the warnings that life can change suddenly, especially when things seem to go well. Coronavirus is a foreshadowing of a future, a warning too. The coronavirus pandemic, if nothing else, already stands as a witness to one of the great lessons that world events can unfold and collapse suddenly. Life as we know it has begun unravelling at the seams and will continue to fall apart for the foreseeable time. Life is tenuous, scary even, but when adding the dimension of an ever-mutating coronavirus, the level of unpredictability rises.

Monday, 30th March
Waiting is an act of surrender

Have you ever sat down and observed the phenomenon of waiting? I know I have not. This is my first. Even though we hardly catalogue its instances, there is plenty of waiting we do in our lifetime. The more I ponder the phenomenon of waiting, it appears to occupy a large share of our daily activities. It fills so much of our lives, yet most of us are oblivious to the lessons it brings. The phenomenon of waiting is best understood as an act of surrender. We often understate it preferring rather to replace it with other less tedious things our favourite pastime. Waiting may be perceived as a hindrance by some, especially people who believe in a full-scale activity calendar with no rest. Because we do not know how to wait, we never to learn how to surrender.

Because we inhabit time with a past and a future, we invariably always wait for something. Why? Because this world is in fact a waiting room. At the end of waiting, there is a faith that we will be able to resuscitate the identifiable routines, which we call life. During our earthly sojourn we are in a season of waiting for one or the other thing. Each wait is individual, it comes in thousand shapes and varieties. We may wait singly or in groups, privately or in community, waiting may be intermittent sometimes it is continuous. Nevertheless, fate binds us to the same end, wait.

I began to consciously make a note of all the reasons people wait. There is no profession that does not have its waiting rooms. All jobs make us waiters. Paid employment entrains much waiting: You have the doctor's waiting rooms when you least can afford to wait given your pain. You wait for the next patient, the next client, the next customer. The delayed airplane, tax refunds, and for the garden to grow. Some long for pathology results to be released like yesterday, some wait for the vaccine to arrive, while others yearn for schools to open again.

There is a classic example of waiting in a checkout line at the Pick n Pay Hyper. There will be several minutes before you get to the cashier, and since there is nothing else to do, you take out your phone and start scrolling through social media feeds. You do not find anything of great interest, after two minutes you put the damn thing back in your pocket and wait for your turn to say 'hi' to the now tired cashier.

We know the feeling of waiting while the phone is plugged on the charger and now there is nothing to do but sit and wait for it to reach that critical 20% before you are able to make that urgent call to your loved one. For the computer message on the screen to pass from 'connecting' to 'connected in a poor network area.' You wait for the slow walker to catch up on a walk; for a fever to abate. Food takes time to cook. Your kids take time to bloom. Love takes time to grow. The first 1000 days of an unborn child to come to term and then for her to start her first tentative step towards walking demands to wait.

We wait in lines at the market to buy theatre tickets, at the bank, coffee houses. For the email response to an application you submitted after you left your last job. For someone to admit they were wrong, or say they love you, for the end of a prison sentence. For the end of everything. Reading this chapter is an exercise of waiting – you are waiting for me to get to the point. You ask, what is the point of this long-winded description of obvious things instead of going to the point, then you jump to the last two chapters for the conclusion of the story? 'I don't have time for this' is a familiar refrain I hear often. The list ends only when life does. Life takes time to unfold.

I rediscovered people watching. People watching has always been a fun and fascinating activity. Plus, I gain valuable insight into the idiosyncratic behaviour of others. Over time, I was able to identify several visual cues. Watching my fellow line-members, I became aware of how people acted depending upon their personality, the environment in which they were, and the other people in line with them. People conveyed a wide range of nonverbal communications while standing in line.

As I observed, some definite patterns of behaviour can be isolated and described. Active, and resigned. Of course, every person is different and may demonstrate any number of the cluster of behaviours. Kami is an active queuer. He demonstrates few common behaviours, including leaning to the side to peer around the line; rocking his body back and forth; turning and looking around the area. He often asks people around him, 'is this queue moving, why don't they open up more lines?' This is not a question he wants answer for, rather he is looking to start a conversation.

Kami never wastes time to move up as openings appears in the line. This guy is usually animated, conversing with the one next or behind him creating a bubble as he moves along the line. He often involves others around him directly in discussions. Depending on the topic of their exchange, most of those around Kami often hear the discussion, invite themselves in and away the circle grows. Usually, but not always, the group along the line never moves congenially. Such is the anatomy of lines.

Tsogo is the typical resigned queuer. While waiting in the queue, she feels stressed by how long the line is. She is resentful to queue for any length of time. *Why don't these Dudes create an app for us to talk to them like I do with everyone else these days*? She wants to abandon the queue, but that would be foolish, Saturday is the only day available, and she cannot change it. However, she does not know what exactly she wants to change. So, she directs her attention towards her shiny iPhone 12.

But once she grabs her phone, another desire appears, this time in the form of finding something interesting to read not to look at. This is another undirected desire with no purpose, so boredom acts as the driving force behind Tsogo's search.

It is when she is longing for something better, without knowing what that better thing might look like. As a result, she tries to satisfy it with a few distractions. She looks to the next thing to alleviate her restlessness but without any purposeful pursuit, the cycle of boredom deepens.

In a way, boredom is inescapable. It acts as the impetus to action, but after that action is complete, it inevitably rears its head again. Avoiding it is largely a futile endeavour, as it is embedded deeply into the human condition.

Our technologies were not meant to take something from us, but they have. We have become a people obsessed with what is speedy and swift, what is immediate. Today Tsogo is reminded that life is not Instagram. Under conditions of lockdown, life is a slow grinding process. Developing only in hours rather than minutes.

My waiting for retirement, does not prescribe the spot in which I stand or even what I shall do at a moment. Many things over which I have no control like the arrival of The Big Day, for example require nothing of me, except that I wait and do not get myself in a position that will disqualify me from collecting the reward in the fulness of time.

Often, waiting is hard and confusing. It seems the lines are always blurred when one come to discern between an instance of a delayed event and one waiting for it to happen. When our lives are put in a holding pan, we complain bitterly and will do everything possible to get things going again. Our way. At its core, impatience is a greater symptom of the real problem—trust. We do not trust the system and the processes. Especially, we do not the freaking government. While I jump at the opportunity to scream 'yes, I trust,' my actions don't tell the same story. Waiting serves an important purpose, revealing our trust in the timing of things. God is at work in our waiting. We might not see any changes in these times of waiting, but there is a purpose after all.

By giving yourself the space to do nothing, you cease looking outwards for novel experiences, and look inwards to uncover the meaning that can be found within your mind. No matter who you are, waiting is an integral part of human life. You will not cease cooling your heels until your soul has lost its warm body. When all the waiting is over, so will be your life.

If we find waiting for the mundane difficult, then waiting on God is even more onerous. What if the waiting room of life is God's design? In his infinite wisdom, God has designed humans for the waiting game. His best classroom for teaching something important to humans who always seem to be in a run for something.

What if, in the waiting the Lord draws us near and imparts lessons we could miss otherwise? Waiting is one of God's tools for developing innate attributes in us. God can see things that need to be ironed out and would only remain creased and messy if it wasn't for the refining times of waiting. In this time, we soon learn that all waiting has a purpose. The best places to meet God is in the between time. The time being is, in a sense, the most trying time of all.

God uses a powerful language of silence. The absence of words reveals much. It is how God use it that reveals its intention, to magnify what already is there. We learn to understand this language when our senses are quietened. This language lacks any phonetic structure, but the way God uses it reveal more about us than words can ever tell. Silence is all about context. 'Be still and know that I am God.' God admonishes the impatient.

What do we do when it seems God is doing nothing? Dead quiet. When we wait it usually implies hanging on until God changes our circumstances. From our perspective we have everything figured out and we want God to fit in our circumstances and on our time, because of this attitude our waiting is more painful than it ought to have been. The trouble, God seldom is in a hurry to do anything.

God uses the waiting time to transform our inner being, a way of smoothing off the rough edges. Instead, God often allows our circumstances to stay the same to a point of almost consuming us while he waits for us to change. God changes us in the throes of our circumstances and not the other way around. God wants us to appreciate things because the longer we must wait for them produces anticipation and we tend to cherish and treasure the things waiting for.

Waiting often reveals our true motive. A lot of what we want to accomplish is to massage our out-sized egos. People who have a bad motive will not wait long because they are not interested in the commitment it takes to see something through. They are invested only in the short-term gains. Waiting surrenders the ego at the altar of silence.

It is not surrender when we are unaware of the waiting, when we do not feel the burn of waiting. Surrender is a virtue so rare and divine that God defines it as the art. Surrendering patiently is the companion of humility. Surrender is the enemy of pride. It was this observation that prompted the author of Ecclesiastes to write, 'the patient in spirit is better than the proud in spirit.'

I like this verse Peter uses, '...The Lord is not slow in keeping his promise, as some understand slowness. Instead, he is patient with you, not wanting anyone to perish, but everyone to come to repentance" (2 Peter 3:8-9).

Our self-centred world has conditioned to have it instantly, almost always. First it was instant coffee and fast food, then it is everything else as well. It is about time we learn what it means to wait and how to do it well. The problem is that our perspective is usually wrong. We tend to think the bigger things in life are possessions, while God thinks loving him and loving people is more important.

In her book, *Seasons of Waiting*, Betsy Howard writes, 'you see, for God, the goal of this school is not that I should learn my lesson so that I don't have to wait anymore.

God wants me to learn how to wait so that I can wait well, even if my waiting continues for the rest of my life. While my plan is to keep a chipper attitude and show God that I am a good student so he will bring my circumstances to a close.

I do not recall who was it that said, 'patience is not the ability to wait but the ability to keep a positive attitude while waiting.' God wants something even better for me. Rather than end my waiting, he wants to educate me in my waiting. My waiting is meant to be a witness not only to myself, but to the watching world.'

The eagle retains his vigour to a great age; and that, he moults in his old age, and renews his feathers, and with them his youth. The winds will blow their freshness into you, and the storms their energy. Your cares and tension will drop away like the leaves of autumn because God renews you in the depth of waiting. The summons to patiently surrender in tribulation is followed by the reward of youthful energy and strength.

We meet the prophet Isaiah where he says, 'even the youth shall faint and be weary, and the young men shall utterly fall, but those who wait upon the Lord shall renew their strength.' Even the youths - such as are in the prime of their strength and glory in it, the most vigorous young men, those in whom we expect manly strength, and who are best suited to endure hardy toil. They become weary through work; their powers are soon exhausted. The most vigorous must be worn down by fatigue or immobilised by sickness, but that the powers of God never grow weary, and that those who trust in him can never become weak.

Yet when the hand of God is upon you, shall grow stronger in faith, patience, and fortitude. Isaiah is telling us the kind of waiting that renews strength is active, not passive. It is a deliberate exchange of human effort for divine strength. Some waiting, far from being burdensome, may be actively cultivated enjoying the journey to our goal, and its million steps, for their own sake. And it is an echo of the unparalleled power and grace of God, 'who acts for those who wait for him.' God asks his people to wait upon him because he is the one who acts for them. And as we bide our time on this side, we keep ourselves in the love of God by 'waiting for the mercy of our Lord Jesus Christ that leads to eternal life.' See Jude 21.

We may not always understand why we must wait, but the good news is that God never asks us to wait without him present. Those who learned their success in life were directly proportionate to their intimacy and dependency upon God. Waiting during the difficult times develops an intimate relationship with God. In the end, they enjoyed the process with God and the promises of God.

God does not leave us alone in the waiting room of life but uses this season of waiting to draw us unto himself. God does not minimize our present painful waiting, rather he fortifies the waiter and lights up the waiting with his presence. Waiting throws a wrench into our coping mechanisms bringing us to the end of our wits because there is nothing we can control. This forces us to rest upon God, the Rock of Ages.

In the New Testament we read in Matthew where Jesus says, 'come to me, all who are weary and heavy burdened, and I will give you rest.' There it is. The waiting room of life is the place where we find rest for our souls not by ourselves but in him. Jesus also gave a lengthy discourse on why believers have no need to worry about anything in their waiting saying, 'don't worry about your life … look at the birds and the lilies.' To a person who is in Christ, worry should be as impossible as it is for birds and flowers, both of which are incapable of anxiety.

In this context, ours is to persevere in our state to the end literally fixing our eyes upon God who provide our refuge. The call is to stand firm in waiting, knowing he will take care of us. Whatever we face and are forced go through, the Lord is there, and we are in his caring arms. When we realise this fact, we can persevere through anything.

Ntombi's husband, a factory worker in his early sixties, has been laid off because her company has closed. They are not financially ready for retirement, but there is no other place likely to employ a pensioner. They are praying to God to provide the husband with a new job, but they do not know when that might be.

Nthabiseng and her husband are both eager for a baby. It is taking longer than she would like to conceive. She has a history of thyroid problem a factor that will affect her ability to conceive. She does not know whether her longing for a baby will stretch on for years or whether her next pregnancy will be soon. She is willing to wait but is she comfortable in the waiting?

Cathy has cerebral palsy. She has been relatively independent for most of her life, but now she is wheelchair bound and has recurring problems with a wound on her foot that will not heal. She spends her time consulting different doctors, none of whom have been able to cure her debilitating wound. Can she confidently wait upon God?

These three people are faced with different situations, but they are each waiting for something. Two are waiting for healing and an end to pain. One is waiting for a job or a business deal. Each kind of waiting shines light on a different facet of the story. None of them know how long their waiting will last. They become students in the school of waiting.

If these characters had suppressed their pain and put on a happy face, they would be missing the deep bass notes that give the gospel such sweet resonance. If there are no tears, then the promise that God 'will wipe away every tear from their eyes' would be a lie. God gives us the opportunity to live out a story that portrays the gospel and serve a kingdom parable.

※ ※

Dear God, you remain the same yesterday, today to eternity. I have searched the Scripture concerning your immutability. I know your tender mercy, wondrous love and unbounded compassion are given to all creation, a gift that is available even to my generation. Merciful Father, you have searched my heart; you know I am neither fearful nor indifferent to the pandemic and its adverse impact on our lives.

As many are bravely making effort to mend their broken lives, to them you seem to have walked off the world stage and abandoned your people to their fate. Others have querulous words, questioning why you allowed this disease to kill their loved ones. Others still have treated the event with indifference declaring, 'if we must die, so be it.'

God, the omnipresent, transcendent, and immanent one, you are the only one who can give answers to the questions this event raises. God, speak now your servant is listening. Speak that I may declare your Word to a nation driven into hopelessness. That I may turn their fears and anxieties into hope. I wait upon you even as I lament the pandemic.

For centuries lament has been the key voice of people in pain, but it remains an unfamiliar method of engagement to the people of this generation. Lament is the language of loss as we grieve together, a language to weep with those who weep. It is the language of loss that should be prayed together as we bring our sorrow to God. Lament provides a language that anchors the grieving people to what they know to be true while they wait.

Lament enters the complicated space of deep disappointment and lingering hurt. Lament is the honest cry of a hurting heart wrestling with the paradox of pain and the promise of God's goodness. Without lament, the people will not know how to process their pain. Even creation groans in times like these. God groans as well.

Lament invites those who are sick in their souls to turn to the author of healing. Without lament, people cannot walk through sorrow. Lament helps us to navigate the wilderness of our grief without going through trite platitudes. Without this sacred song of sorrow, it is easy to miss the lessons historic lament is intended to teach us. There is a song of mercy to be sung under dark clouds. The space between brokenness and God's mercy is where a song is sung, it is the path from heartbreak to hope. Lament invites us to turn our gaze from the rubble of life to the redeemer of it.

Confusion, but especially exhaustion, can cause us to retreat from the one who knows our sorrows. The mist of bitterness can sweep in, creating a fog of unbelief and a justification for our behaviour. Even though hope feels distant, lamenters reach out to God through hardship. Godly lamenters keep asking even when the answer is delayed. Lament talks to God, seeking his mercy.

Lament candidly talks to God about what is wrong. It vocalises circumstances that do not seem to fit with God's character or his purposes. While we know God is in control, there are times in our limited human vision when it feels like God has absented himself in the world stage. When it seems that injustice rules the day, lament invites us to talk to God about it. All suffering has an expiration date. It will not last forever you too, will get past it. Lament helps us through suffering by directing our hearts hidden behind the pain.

Lament gives us permission to verbalise the tension. And the more honest we can be, the sooner we are able to move to the next element. Laments are poems set to music;

this framework provides the structure for talking to God about the brokenness of the world we live in.

Lament seeks more than belief; it yearns for the deliverance that fits with God's character. Lament affirms the applicability of God's promises by asking again and again for help. But also encourages us to embrace the final point of all lament: a renewal of trust. Confidence in God's trustworthiness is the ultimate destination of all laments.

Our usual response to the relational pain is to push away the story that God has permitted in our lives (pain) that inevitably leads to some bitterness but by receiving the cup that God has permitted in our lives, we neuter the evil we take the cup offered to us by God, so the evil one can no longer capture our soul.

At the apex of the first wave of the coronavirus pandemic I heard cries from Italy, *Tutto entire bene*, meaning 'all will go well.' A mantra to exorcise the worries from their minds. This Italian slogan was found in blog posts, pictures, and messages that Italians exchanged with frenzy. The hope that all will go well was grounded in the promises of therapeutic medicine curing the sick and in science to find a vaccine. All will go well can be misleading if it is not grounded in the theology of God, the hope of our glory.

For all its wonderful achievements, even science will capitulate to the inexorability of death. Medicine is not our ultimate hope—God is. Science is not our ultimate resource—God is. Without recognizing the God of the Bible as the God of everything, they hoped-for happy conclusion to this pandemic and to all crises is misplaced hope. Fear will continue to have the last word.

During the plague in his era, Martin Luther applied these words, 'I shall ask God to protect us mercifully. Then I shall fumigate, help purify the air, administer medicine, and take it. I shall avoid places and persons where my presence is not needed in order not to become contaminated and thus perchance pollute others and so cause their death because of my negligence.

If God should wish to take me, he will surely find me, and I have done what he has expected of me and so I am not responsible for either my own death or the death of others. If my neighbour needs me, however, I shall not avoid place or person but will go freely. See, this is such a God-fearing faith because it is neither brash nor foolhardy and does not tempt God.'

The pandemic is not a historical or personal blip that interrupted our lives. It is a cataclysmic event involving more loss than we know, and it set us on a new path. The old path is gone. And until we fully grieve what we have lost, we will not be able to make sense of what is new. Rosie Spinks talks of grieving, 'holding space for everything I've lost is precisely what has allowed me to create something entirely new with my life this year. Once I started examining what I had lost, honouring it, and allowing it, I started to see all the other ways my life needed to change to adapt to what's coming.

There are any number of ways to grieve, but the simplest is to just give yourself the time and space to consider all you have been through this year. Set aside few minutes a day to sit in a quiet room and notice how you feel. Allow the feelings you usually avoid arising. Do not judge them when they do. Ritualize it.

Make it a part of your new life because it is ultimately a positive force. When you make adequate time and space to honour your grief and feel it move through your body, things start to happen. Grief, if you cede to it, can serve as an embodied reminder that what we are all doing here is a one-time limited offer. The only certainty is that it is going to end. It is the ultimate 'memento mori.' Grief is not a situational balm, rather it is a healthy practice. We may need it now more than ever, but we always will.

Thursday, 30th March
Maar, what is this thing?

Nowhere does brooding winter sky shakes quiet like the Northwest. I looked across the open estuary of the Magalies river, pale yellow sunlight filtered through streaks of low-lying cloud, reflected in the mirror-like ribbons of water and ripples of sand exposed by the retreating tide. All around, fields dipped gently to flatten out along the never-ending berg, which snakes its way westwards to the mining towns of Mogale city and beyond.

The lowland, flanked by rolling hills, expands until the berg meets the dam, creating a natural break in the land between Magaliesberg and Broederstroom. The area around Magaliesberg spreads like one vast prairie. Here, the winds blow bitter cold in winter; the sun patches the soil in summer and ranchers, farmers, and folks from this 500-people community gather for a weekend pop-up farmers bazaar.

Standing firm against a determined breeze, I stood atop a grassy knoll looking out over a sweep of alien landscape. Set against a gunmetal-grey sky, a rich autumnal carpet was draped over valleys and mountains alike, giving the distant mountain summits a softness as the clouds gathered at their nape. A deep inky pool rippled in the morning light, reflecting the moodiness of the passing sky.

I am in Magalies the wild heartland bordering Gauteng and the Northwest. I am surveying the surroundings that mark the south end border of Gauteng and Northwest. Peacefully admiring nature at work. It is hard to believe that this seemingly tranquil rural landscape was once at the edge of one of South Africa's bloodiest wars. Today, this once troublesome region is laid back and a quiet part of the border where hardy animal breeds are reared, and a sense of community reverberates among the established households.

This lesser visited part of Gauteng is also where I get to know it intimately. A place where local histories and scant ruins linger among the wooded valleys, fast-flowing rivers and open moorland that lend themselves to letting my imagination fill some blanks of its much-under-told story. The wild, often barren landscape, punctuated only by hills and plains, adds to the effect.

Magalies river ran just over eight kilometres across at its widest, and roughly 33 kilometres from the elevated north down to the sandy-flats of the west with Fourways at its south-western tip and around one third of the area extending into the north eastern Pretoria. Magalies also proved perfectly placed as a launching pad for my foray, only a brief detour from the N14. The architecture reflects the early 20th century well, such as the once-upon-a-time colonial revival-style life whose adjoining café I was thawing out in.

Magalies has an appeal for the farming community; the intrigue of this unfathomable period and, by association, the surrounding villages of Broederstroom, whose natural landscapes remain almost as wild and untamed as in the days of the colonial era. This farming community is tranquil until the topic of coronavirus is broached to one of its residents then it changes its complexion.

I am at the annual bazaar where I farm produce is sold in an open market. After packing my Ostrich stake, Macadamia nuts and three bags of Gemsbok biltong into the carry bag, he thought I was done. He proceeded to place his goodies on the table. I shifted to the side while watching him shuffle the merchandise one after the other on the counter of stall number seven. Our eyes met momentarily, I smiled, a warm flush rising from the base of my neck to my temples and while standing still. He realised the error of his way and self-corrected at once.

'I am sorry, my senior moment right there, I did not realise you are not done yet. Please, go ahead finish your shopping.' He says sheepishly.

I gave him the biggest smile reserved only for my fiancé Ayo in pre-coital moments.

'No worries, don't we all have our moments.'

'Much appreciated. Thank you, Sir.'

He opened his wallet and took out a R200 note to finalise his purchase, the man behind the table shook his head three times.

'No change, Sir.'

'Here, take this.' I spoke. He extends his hand taking my notes, one R100 and two R50s. He raises his left finger motioning me to wait for him while he collects the change from the stall keeper. He appeared keen to speak to me about what, I don't know. I wait on the side as I have been.

He is a middle-aged man, pale with liquid eyes, standing there with a smile. I do not think the reason he noticed me was because I was the only Afrikan mingling amongst a largely Afrikaner community at a farm produce shandy. His curiosity went beyond the mundane. He starts by sussing out randomly innocuous information not with any goal in mind.

'What brings you around here, are you a local man?'

'I live on the other side of town, I regularly come to the craft market. I love the organic products they make here. I am thinking of becoming a vegan sometime in the future.' I lied.

'Wow, nice to know.'

'What about you?' Fixing my gaze on his sun-drenched face.

'I am part-time farmer and a university teacher.'

'Our stall is over there, pointing at the opposite side of the bazaar; I would like to show you what we grow in our farm. We have organically cultured maas and honey.

He leads me to the far end where the bazaar is less congested.

I caught the bit about university teaching and lurched onto it. I learn that he trains infectious diseases scientists at the university, I also learn he knows something about the current pandemic outbreak that has gone from one country to the rest of the world.

In my curiosity, I lurch onto this and pursue it gently hoping he would not fluster under pressure and seek refuge to something less intrusive or just dump me there. I threw in a fishing question of my own. 'What are the characteristics of coronavirus and why is it so infectious so much so that some of those who are infected by it are killed within four weeks while others recover from the infection in eleven days yet, another population group never show any symptoms at all?'

He took me to a nearby willow tree. Large. The branches were hanging low into a river below. There was a big log straddling the tree and the river embankment steady enough to be a temporary stool for the two of us. He watched me fumble with the buckle of my sling leather bag hanging across my shoulders, he glanced sideways while waiting for me to settle my ruffled ass down. He removed his glasses to wipe his eyes. He is soft spoken, not rushed in his speech and erudite in presentation.

'Do you mind my asking what interest brings you to the area of infectious disease?'

'I see patients every day, I'd like to be armed with up to date information when I dispense advise to them.' I said plainly.

'Glad to know. Let us get down to it then, shall we!'

'The story goes something like this, some random Chinese folk was shopping for the usual at the seafood market at Huanan, because it's a big place to walk through at some point he got hungry and decided to sample a soup made from bat meat. Now the Americans are paying for his plate.'

I laughed out aloud nearly fell off the wooden log. His chuckle remains somewhat guarded. He returned to my question anyway.

It was 3 January 2020, and Supaporn Wacharapluesadee was standing by, awaiting a delivery at her lab. Word had spread that there was respiratory disease affecting people in Wuhan, and with the Lunar New Year approaching, many Chinese tourists were headed to neighbouring Thailand to celebrate. Cautiously, the Thai government began screening passengers arriving from Wuhan at the airport, and a few select labs were chosen to process the samples to try to detect the problem.

Wacharapluesadee is an expert virus hunter. Over the past 10 years, she is part of Predict, an organisation that detect and stop diseases that can jump from non-human animals to humans. She and her team's main focus has been on bats, which are known to harbour many coronaviruses.

Although China notified the world health organisation of the known cluster case of coronavirus[1] on the evening of December 31, 2019, it is believed the earliest date is around November 17, 2019. Coronavirus is a pathogen that is stripped down to the essentials of information and reproduction. On January the 6th systems around the world, began to activate their incident management protocols. Not long afterwards, on the 15th January, China typed the genetic sequence of the coronavirus to help provide information to scientists across the globe in responding to the new virus.

The pathogen evolved in the great big ocean of wildlife, some spread to farm animals, some contaminate drinking water, some get a host in mosquito, cow, camel, pig, birds, and dogs. You can even find viruses in the soil.

The influence of viruses on life on earth goes far beyond the tragedies of a single species. Then they found the human body to be a hospitable host and are learning to settle inside. Even though we know that two thirds of all infectious diseases come from animals, we have lived with viruses for thousands of years without major health complications like we are experiencing today.

Coronaviruses are a large family of different viruses and have been around the earth for as long as animals have lived and are not dangerous. The coronavirus is not new in the world, neither is it new to humans. Circa 6th century AD the first coronavirus was circulating in Wuhan, China. Although the virus does not make animals sick, it makes humans sick that is why it is has the prefix novel. They are known to have infected bats, camels, and cattle. Coronavirus cause most of the colds that affect us during the winter season but do not pose serious threat to the health of humans nor indeed complicate the functioning of our bodies to a point of death.

Epidemiologists from the world health organisation have begun their work to figure out if indeed the coronavirus outbreak's epicentre was Wuhan's wet market where wild animals were killed on the spot and sold to waiting customers or was it brought there through other agents. Because of the similarities in their genetic material this has made it uncertain which animal exactly is responsible. Therefore, scientists are still working to confirm if the virus SARS-nCOV-2 jumped from a bat to a pangolin or some intermediary before it jumped to humans through aerosolization.

In 1960 virologists discovered that Coronavirus is not one but a group of viruses that belong to the family of *Coronaviridae*. Since then scientists have divided coronaviruses into seven families with sub-groups called alpha, beta, gamma, and delta. Seven of these sub-groups can infect humans, which are 299E (alpha), NL63 (alpha), OC43(beta) and HKU1 (beta). The less known are MERS-COV, a beta virus that causes Middle East Respiratory Syndrome (MERS), Sudden Acute Respiratory Syndrome (SARS COV, a beta virus that causes SARS-nCOV-2 which causes COVID-19 disease. All viruses change over time due to the phenomenon of genetic mutation.

---

[1] Quotations on the coronavirus are extracted from the sources in the reference section, which are cited in the endnotes.

It was the World Health Organisation that identified this new type of coronavirus and gave it its name novel Severe Acute Respiratory Syndrome Coronavirus (SARS-nCOV-2) the virus that causes COVID-19 the disease that complicates the entire body to a point of death. According to WHO this virus is a new human pathogen.

As frightening as it is coronavirus is not a living organism but a genetic particle with some membrane type of coat on them. To simplify it, this virus is a fleck of DNA wrapped in a lockpick bag of proteins. It cannot reproduce on its own without using the cellular machinery of a living host. Until it enters a human host where it attaches itself with its tentacles to cell and make many copies of itself inside the cell, otherwise outside its host it dies naturally. It is harmless on its own. This virus does not have energy, because it does not do anything it neither creates nor uses energy. It has no metabolism; it is biologically inert. It just sits there, anywhere. On a surface, it remains effective for three days until washed off.

The coronavirus is not visible at any wavelength of light human can perceive. You need a powerful magnifying electron microscope to see it, this thing is around 0.07 microns. Think of it in relation to a strand of human hair diameter which is 75 microns, then you know it is an infinitesimally small thing we are talking about.

'If I think of it as a speck of dust am I closer to imagining it?'

'Not by a long, short. A speck of dust you can see with your naked eye or in my case with glasses, this shit is invisible. Period.'

He trained his eyes on me sizing up my reaction to his word choice. eKasi this is how we talk; I am not shocked by it. Stone-faced, I just nodded to his forthrightness.

'Coronavirus has 5 million atoms in its coat and 60 thousand atoms in its genome. Changing any one of them causes the virus to behave in new ways. Mutation is a random change not planned or controlled by the virus itself but manipulated by nature, hence the complexity in figuring effective countermeasures.

Straining his neck, he looked up in the sky, blaming the clouds for cold breeze hitting our faces. This time his smile seemed fake, but his eyes sparkled with warmth and re-assuring. He pulls out two sticks of sun-dried, per-peri Gemsbok biltong from a brown bag sitting between his legs he offers me one while he smells his before chomping it in half. 'matured in the shade 30-days I guess?' I say. He nods in agreement.

'Although the virus was discovered in China sometimes late November 2019, he continues, we don't know for sure if it originally came from there and for how long it has been circulating. What made things difficult the virus was hidden by a long incubation period. The Chinese have not found Patient Zero, which is critical to us scientists in determining the origins of this thing. The earliest known patient had not visited Huanan Seafood Market for months before the first case was reported in Wuhan.

We know it spread to other parts of the world in the early weeks of January 2019. My suspicions are it could have been in China much earlier than we thought. The virus spread through person-to-person contact what is now commonly known as community transmission. This happens through breathing, coughing, and sneezing. It may have started with the infected person coughing or sneezing saliva droplets amid closed quarters. The virus got out through the droplets coughed or from the surfaces that others touched then touching their faces afterwards.

Countries outside China made the same mistake first made by China (excerpt for Taiwan) of thinking 'this thing was not contagious we will have it under control in no time. We have first world public health care system that we can mobilise and deploy at scale.' Where leaders believed in their own invincibility, I can safely say hubris more than the virus killed people in those countries. We know this is true of the Americas but especially the USA.

Coronavirus emerged in a human population from a combination of factors; zoonotic transmission that is, a virus jumping from an animal to humans and the formation of human reservoir where the virus needs to spread between humans. Crowded conditions can let the virus triumph.

The disease normally shows in a person infected between 2 and 14 days by developing pneumonia, respiratory failure, septic shock, or death. Coronavirus can only be viewed in a rear-view mirror: by the time a person becomes a patient, that critical moment of transmission has already happened.

In the early stages something like two weeks after infection the body's immune system respond with symptoms like a sore throat, a fever or dry cough loss of smell and taste and shortness of breath. If the body fails to rid itself of the infection, the virus moves down to into the respiratory tract and stomach. The virus latches its spiky surface proteins to receptors on the surface of the epithelial cells in our body.

ACE2 receptors are found in epithelial cells throughout the body. The lower airways have more of these receptors and so COVID-19 attaches easily and makes millions of copies of itself rapidly. Once inside the cell, it blocks distress signal proteins that the cell makes when under attack, it also destroys antiviral commands inside infected cells this gives the virus time to make very many copies in a short space of time and infect surrounding cells before the body's immune system identifies it as an invader. Therefore, the virus can spread before the fever begin to show up in the symptoms.

But when the body cannot destroy the virus at its entry point, viral particles go deeper inside the body where it can take a few paths setting up camp in the lungs or go to the digestive tract often-times going both ways at the same time. Once it is embedded in the body, it begins to cause severe illness. In all patients infected with COVID-19 the symptoms vary from loss of appetite, diarrhoea, indigestion, pinkeye and loss of smell and taste to developing severe respiratory complications as seen in the shortness of breath.

This may be the reason for the vast array of symptoms COVID-19 can cause. The more the virus is in such areas the more inflammation is seen in the area. Severe damage to the lungs may be one trigger that activates the immune system to release a barrage of chemicals known as cytokines.

The sudden flood of these chemicals is called cytokines storm, it is the body's reaction to defend itself against the invading virus. This chemical overreaction causes blood pressure to drop which sets off the rapid onset of abnormally low levels of oxygen in the blood also known as hypoxia and it is the reason for sudden decompensation in the body leading to critical illness in COVID -19 patients. Put simply, it is not the coronavirus that kills the patient *per se*, but the body's hyper-reaction to its invasion in the form of uncontrolled production of pro-inflammatory cytokines.

If patient's system can combat viral replication with some efficiency due to their age, genetics, and other indices of immune competence the patient will have a lower set point. Could a lower initial exposure, also lead to a lower set point? Faced with this challenge, the immune system could have a greater chance of controlling the pathogen.

In contrast, if a person is inundated with multiple high-dose exposures, the swiftly replicating invader could gain ground that the immune system might be hard-pressed to conquer. Now we know from clinical data that from first day of infection including the incubation period to time of death the patient has four weeks to clear the virus or surely will die. The longer the patient is on the ventilator – we have estimated from clinical data that three weeks or longer - the less are the chances of that patient's recovery.

There is another aspect of transmission and disease however, the host immune response. Viral attack and the immune system's defence are two opposing forces constantly fighting. What was the total 'force' of the microbial presence? What host factors was limiting the microbial invasion i.e. genetics, prior exposure to the same virus, baseline immune competence? And then was the initial equilibrium tipped towards the virus, or towards the host? The immune system makes antibodies to track down and kill the coronavirus clones that has hijacked the cell and their machinery to make more copies of itself.

Around 8-10 days after the initial symptoms have shown, the infected person has shortness of breath and the condition deteriorates to acute respiratory distress syndrome a few days later. This syndrome damages the tissues and blood vessels in the tiny air sacs causing debris to collect inside them.

This makes it harder to breathe the infected person must be sedated, intubated, connected onto a ventilator to breathe for them. If not put on the oxygen it means the lungs are not supplying the vital organs with enough oxygen causing them to shut down one-by-one and eventually stop working causing the cessation of the heart function.'
Tulio pauses and smile at me as if to invite me to challenge his assertions.

'What about temperature levels, is the virus more potent or less so depending on the heat gauge?'

'The virus is stable between 4-6 degrees Celsius; it is also stable at room temperature. It converts to non-infectious after 90 minutes of exposure at 56 degrees.'

'Ambient heat is the virus chief enemy it cannot not survive it.'

'And so, between the 10th and 18th June and between the 7th and 17th July, the two coldest periods of our winter we have seen more people contract the virus and more deaths in the aftermath compared to the other time during the pandemic. If you are looking for your positive correlation, there it is right there.'

He speaks with authority and clarity of mind like a man who works as an Epidemiologist. I could not hide the fact that I am super impressed with his knowledge and the sense of awe at his depth. I give it to him.

'I can tell you are a knowledgeable Scientist and am in awe of your knowledge.'

'Do you perhaps work in a virology laboratory or something.'

'I work as Epidemiologist and Teacher of postdoctoral researchers at Wits university.'

'Wow, it's easy to tell from your knowledge. You have piqued my interest in the subject of coronavirus. I also know that you are busy at the craft market with your stall and everything. Do you mind if we continue this discussion on some other day when you are more available?'

'What's your station in life?'

With this question, I figured he wanted me to confirm his suspicion, I ignored it by diverting attention to the more functional aspect of my engagement with him.

'Do you have email address that I can use to arrange time to progress this discussion?' At first, he appeared hesitant, perhaps miffed at my insolence, I cannot be certain. Somehow he what changed his mind.

'Sure, here is my card. I'll be happy to take you through the science that seek to respond to the pandemic.'

I was surprised to watch him shake hands with me, nevertheless he did. We parted ways, each to his own. I walk through the remaining farm stalls checking merchandise to take home. I made sure to remember as much detail as I had managed to take in during this rich encounter. Rare.

A quick Google search reveals several interesting clues about the stature and accomplishments of this diminutive man. Tulio de Guerra is a Professor of Medicine specialising in Epidemiology at the Wits School of Medicine. He is also current Director of the South African Centre for Epidemiological Modelling and Analysis. His research interests focus on emerging, zoonotic, and vector-borne pathogens. A Visiting Research Fellow in Tropical Disease Modelling at UCL, London. He is a published author of several peer-reviewed papers in leading academic journals.

※ ※

Two days later, I sent Tulio a short email thanking him for our chat and expressed a need to meet with him again. A day later I was included in the mailing list to a briefing session due on Thursday of the same week to a select audience of Epidemiologists, post-Doctoral Researchers, and a regular clientele of practising physicians. I had to re-organise my work schedule to free up the time for an afternoon I would not want to miss.

I was on the money; his talk was a longer version of the WHO updates only his was rich with anecdotal stories and insightful observations. He presented to us the symptoms, current treatment regime and vaccine research work his consortium collaborates with global agencies.

I came early to meet him first but also curious to check out his research centre. Where he works there is a large auditorium where invited guest filed in. During the greet-and-meet session pre-talk, Tulio appears light-hearted telling us anecdotal stories from the townships and suburbs. He jumped to the mountain of power point slides he has prepared pointing this or that to us. It was difficult to know when he started with the presentation proper or when he was still fooling around with jokes, in any case I caught up with him at the point where he was saying.

'Up until now, there is no vaccine, monoclonal antibodies (mAbs), or drugs available to treat the disease. In most people infected with the coronavirus the immune system is quite capable of dealing with the virus so that they do not get sick, among those who do the immune system eventually rids the body of the virus and the patient recover on his own. The recovery rate of around 86% of the population.

A small number of those infected who present comorbidities needed hospitalisation. Once hospitalised, most received IV fluids and oxygen or get linked to ventilators to help them breathe. Of hospitalised patient population, a small number cannot be helped they die. The mortality rate is generally lower than 3.5% of the population if that at all.

Coronavirus it seems is relatively stable. It acquired about two mutations a month in the eight months of spreading. Nevertheless, this necessitated the WHO to update the warning signs of the coronavirus. Based on a review of more than 1000 patients who have already sought care Harvard Medical School researchers offered a new list of symptoms to be included in the case definition.

Fever is not a reliable indicator of COVID-19. Often people who show up at hospital ERs with respiratory symptoms have only slightly elevated body temperatures, COVID-19 may begin with various permutations of cough without fever, sore throat, diarrhoea, abdominal pain, headache, body ache and fatigue. What really sets more serious cases of COVID-19 apart is something that is almost never seen in influenza or other respiratory illness: severe shortness of breath.

Shortness of breath is a feeling that you cannot fill your lungs with air as you normally do. It appears four or more days after onset of other symptoms. Shortness of breath gets worse with physical exertion, including performing simple activities like walking, climbing stairs. Shortness of breath is a really warning sign that a person might need hospitalisation.' Additionally, sense of smell most often diminishes by the 3rd day of infection with coronavirus and many patients also lose their sense of taste, a new study finds.

Some have started talking about this not as a lung disease but a blood disease where the virus attacks directly haemoglobin molecules and affects the oxygen transport. Cardiologists have started to speculate the coronavirus may directly infect the heart because blood vessel cells have the same receptors that damages the blood vessels thus may cause an inflammation of the heart muscle.

Current medical intervention available to treating doctors are post-exposure prophylactic treatment for the admitted patients. The post-exposure prophylactic intervention ensured that the infection was kept mild rather than severe so that patient's immune system could fight the virus and recover on its own.

Doctors began a trial of combination of recovery treatment drugs from the existing stock to see if they can slow down the effects of the virus in the body. Antivirals aimed at limiting the spread of the coronavirus inside the body were the obvious candidates. While immune system modulators limited the damage, the body does to itself while fighting off the virus.

A cocktail of antiviral drugs has been tried by doctors in various jurisdictions. In USA for example they tried the combinations of *Arbidol/favipiravir/baloxavir* drugs to treat flu to see if it can help patients recover fast from the coronavirus, this drug however failed the test. Elsewhere doctors used the HIV/Aids combinations of *Lopinavir/Ritonavir/nelfinavir* as a preventative measure. In randomised trials no benefits were shown by these drugs for patients in the ICU. Neither did *Nitazoxanide* show any benefits for the patients suffering from COVID-19.

A successful clinical trial was *Remdesivir* an IV drug used in people with COVID-19 as a potent direct-acting antiviral agent or polymerase inhibitor for coronavirus. Although developed to fight the Ebola infection and used successfully against the MERS virus in the previous outbreak the drug has indeed slowed the COVID-19 progression with improved result from 15 days to 11 days recovery time.

The trial of *hydroxychloroquine* a malaria and arthritis drug failed the trials. *Ribavirin,* a broad-spectrum antiviral used in combination with *Interferon alpha* was also tried, the results remain inconclusive. In a small trial, doctors in Spain tried *Interferon Beta* with great promise, a larger trial results are awaited.

An immune modulating drug *Tocilizumab* treating rheumatoid arthritis was tried, this drug showed a massive benefit in the trial for the severely ill patients. However, in a study by the University of Oxford found the drug *Dexamethasone* had shown to reduce death among patients on oxygen therapy and ventilation by a margin of 30% at 6mg once a day. The study was done in 175 hospitals involving 11,500 patients. This drug has shown to act on modulating the immune system. This drug is also used to treat leukaemia and terminal brain tumours as well as arthritis.

A convalescent plasma therapy to treat the virus using blood serum from recovered patients is spearheaded by John Hopkins group as a means of preventing healthy people notably front-line medical staff, from getting sick or, on patients who are moderately ill to see if the serum will keep them out of ICU and help bring them back to health. Doctors say the treatment will probably serve as a bridge until other drugs and vaccine become available.

Another study used a trial of ARMS-1 antiseptic that patients spray into their mouths 3X a day to reduce the upper respiratory tract infections. This antiseptic spray was used in patients with bone marrow suppression. Several other trials were reported but at the time of this publication no data had been published yet.'

When the virus peaked in this country, its potency would have weakened sufficiently to be less virulent, I hope that though it would still be infectious, it will not kill as much. The reports that came out from Italy confirmed this hypothesis. It is common for virus to be less deadly over time. The reasoning is that if a virus is too deadly for humans to risk an infection, we take measures that hinders the virus from procreating. This introduces high selection pressure, which prefers less deadly strains that would let us lift the measures. We are basically pressurising the virus into becoming less dangerous so that we can simply live with it the same way we do with the flu and common colds.'

'Esteemed colleagues, with six months of research into the behaviour of coronavirus including reviewing tomes of literature around the world, my conclusion come down to a simple fact; do not worry about treatment we don't have any. Advice your patients to eat for immunity.

My opinion is that we do not have to worry so much about the lack of recovery treatment drugs as much as becoming aware that our bodies are perfectly capable of defending themselves from this thing if we keep our immune system strong. Put simply, to ensure we survive COVID-19 we must strengthen our immune system. My sense is that you should take this advice and give it to your patients. The information pack we have prepared contains the guidance you need in full. Let me highlight a few here.

Sleeping well. And of the various ways to boost immunity, the simplest is to get enough sleep. Someday, COVID-19 will be a dim, bygone nightmare, but right now the pandemic remains a useful wakeup call to remind us that good sleep hygiene can help boost our immune systems.

Outdoor life. Getting outdoors does improve the quality of our sleep, that's a given. Our circadian rhythms are usually kept synchronised to the time of the day when we are outdoors. Circadian disruption and sleep curtailment have been linked to a reduced immune system response. Light has a strong impact via its ability to entrain the circadian rhythm and improved sleep. Humans adapt on planet with a 24-hour cycle of light and dark, and our bodies are set up to work in partnership with sunlight. 'Oh, while I am at it, do remind the patients that bright sunlight has a positive impact on their mood too.' There is big laughter in the room.

Eating good food. The following are the kinds of food good for strengthening the immune system. Lots of whole fruits, nuts and seeds including almonds, peanuts, and sunflower seeds. Veggies include sweet potatoes, broccoli, carrots, and spinach. Salmon fish and dairy products can fortify our constitution greatly.

Vitamin D. There is established relationship between the functioning of the innate and adaptive immune system and vitamin D. Immune system that is tops needs a vitamin D blood level of 50 to 80 ng/mL. This daily dose of vitamin D can help to strengthen our bones and teeth, but it also has a direct effect on our immune system. Vitamin D enables the macrophages in our lungs to spew out an antimicrobial peptide called cathelicidin killing viruses directly.

Simplify this by advising patients that spending a minimum of 30 minutes daily preferably in the morning until noon time or before 2pm when the sun's UVB rays are at their peak is the best medicine from mother nature. Sunlight energises special cells in our immune system called B and T-cells that help fight infection. Vitamin D also changes the availability of the same ACE2 receptors on the lung cells. If vitamin D has already altered these receptors, then it may make it harder for the virus to gain a foothold in the body.

The patient can do this by walking in a park, woodland, or other green spaces, then so much better. Numerous studies have shown that getting outdoors in nature lowers people's blood pressure as well as normalising secretion of the stress hormone, cortisol. Walking outside in the woodland has many benefits, trees are affecting our immune system more directly - several studies have suggested that spending a few days in a forest results in an increase in the number of our killer cells that help to detect and destroy viruses in our blood. Plants in the open make phytoncides that when we breath in seem to bolster our immune system too.

Regular aerobic exercise appears to help the body fight illness caused by viruses. That is in part because it helps blood get around the body more efficiently, which means germ-fighting substances get where they need to go. This is true not only for the common flu, but also for Covid-19 coronavirus. These various pathways work in synergy nothing in isolation.

Specialist doctors discourage people from taking OTC immune boosters supplements because supplements tend to undermine the person's natural immune system rather than boost it. One last thing before we take a comfort break. From an epidemiological perspective, our focus has always been less on the number of people who will die due to coronavirus, we look to the living for clues. We are the branch of science that believes science does not prevent death, it merely prolongs life where this is possible.' Tulio concludes his address to a mute applause.

Several hands are held up from the audience in the front and at the back of the auditorium. 'I notice many hands rising; I'll be glad to chat during the break.' He tells his curious doctors in the audience.

We break for tea. A member of staff enters the room carrying a laptop and yanks Tulio's notebook out of the docking station and swaps it around. She plugs it in. Test if it works and with a thumbs up sign the staff shouts, 'we good to go, girl.' The next presenter who was seated among the audience walks up to the podium with thumbs raised in response, without much funfair she walks up to the front and check the presentation herself while the audience are taking time to enjoy sandwiches and scones.

※ ※

'My unit is multi-disciplinary; I am blessed to attract some of the best scientific minds in the field. The next presenter needs little introduction if at all, her published work and community involvement speaks for her accomplishments. She is a pre-eminent scholar in the field of epidemiology. Doctor Nontobeko Ntuli, you can call her Ntobs, she is cool with that, trust me is a Resident Senior Researcher. She will speak to us about the virus's characteristics, pathophysiology in humans and what kinds of vaccines are in the pipeline from the pharma world.

The boss's praise in the presence of pre-eminent scientists, doctors and high-powered philanthropists can be an intoxicating tonic tending to obligate the recipient to reciprocate in kind often over the top. It is not uncommon to hear recipients of praise saying things not meant to be, for example, 'Thank you Professor, for your warm and kind words.

I feel honoured to work for such a prestigious research house and am proud to be associated with household name such as yourself. This organisation is at the cutting edge of research, right up there with the best funded research houses in the world. We know everything that's coming our way, and we are the first to tell it to the world.' She could have said this and more. No. Ntobs chose a different route. In her demeanour she is unpretentious yet comfortable in her own skin. It is almost as if she is saying to Tulio, I got this. Thank you very much but I do not need validation from a man.

Ntobs skips the frills and the polite fiction cutting straight to the chase. 'An article titled "A novel coronavirus outbreak of global health concern" published on the British medical journal *The Lancet* on January 24th indicated the origin of the virus may differ from what was first thought. Seven clinicians from Jinyan hospital, one of the hospitals treating COVID-19 patients in Wuhan, revealed in that paper that 13 of the first 41 cases they had treated had no link to the Huanan Seafood Market, the initial location to which cases of COVID-19 were linked was found between the first patient and later cases.'

'There are virus-infected patients outside of China who had never travelled to or were ever connected with individuals from China. In Paris and California respectively, the first COVID-19 cases were reported in December 2019 from patients who had not travelled outside the USA and France or meeting another patient known to have the infection. Robertfield confirmed that some COVID-19 deaths have been misdiagnosed as flu-related in the USA. Maria Vankerhove, technique lead of WHO Health Emergency programme confirmed the same when she said, 'some early cases did not have exposure at the market. There is a lot of area of work that needs to be conducted to identify the real intermediary hosts.'

With that kind of opening remarks, I sit up and take notice of the speaker. Ntobs possess not only tantalising beauty but also has fun personalities. Her friendly face strikes a chord with her audience. This Durban-born girl arrested my attention – cosy, charming, dressed to perfection. Her hair is chestnut brown. Her noise perfectly straight, narrow, foreshortened, emphasising the provocative fullness of her mouth. Her eyes are set wide apart, big, and rounded like a russet apple. The dimpled pink face beneath the long silky hair is cherubic. Her beatific smile lit up her face and gives her supermodel appeal.

No spot or blemish marred her skin. Her face is a synthesis of perfect symmetry. Her gorgeousness is a matter of minor adjustment to a pattern of girls from Durban. I am transfixed by the perfection of her shoulders and the back of her head. I could have looked at her for hours on end, trying to locate the source of my fascination. She is the *it* girl.

To the question many have asked, 'what makes one healthy person contract the coronavirus and fight for her life on a ventilator in hospital while another gets through the infection almost symptom-free? For that matter, what makes anyone go to the hospital with COVID- 19 when not everyone does?'

The answer is written in our genes. Researchers around the world are trying to find out which ones. As researchers begin to comb the human genome, our estimated 25,000 genes for genes that might play a role in COVID-19 infection, they have a few suspects in mind. Early studies not yet published in peer-reviewed journals suggest that variations in a gene called HLA plays a role. HLA tells the body how to make specific proteins that the immune system uses to recognize intruding germs in the body. These germs are then marked as targets and killed.

Researchers at Oregon Health and Science University suggested that variations in this gene from one person to the next could result in proteins that are better or worse at recognizing and flagging the coronavirus in the body. The researchers checked this theory against previous genetic research in people who had severe acute respiratory syndrome caused by another type of SARS coronavirus during the 2002 outbreak.

The theory tracked people who had certain versions of HLA had more severe SARS infections and more of the virus in their bodies than those with other versions. Only genetic studies in real people who have had COVID-19 can confirm the HLA theory. Researchers are pursuing this with keen interest.

The TMPRSS2 gene is another. This gene also involved in flu infection, helps create a protein that the coronavirus uses to get inside human cells. Some people produce high levels of the protein others less. If research can prove that people who produce less of the protein do much better with COVID-19, 'this would make very clear to us that interfering with TMPRSS 2 would be an important treatment strategy.' says David Goldstein Director of the Columbia University Institute for Genomic Medicine.

Researchers have their eyes on ACE2 as well. This gene helps produce ACE2 receptors on the surface of human cells. The spikey coronavirus plugs its bristles into these ACE2 ports so it can latch onto the cell. So, ACE2 does seem the logical thing to go after in genetic research.

Genetic studies can often have surprise results. Questioning only the suspects makes it possible to miss scores of other accomplices. When Goldstein and his colleagues looked for genes that play a part in hepatitis C infection years ago, he says, everyone had their favourite candidate genes they were looking at IL 28 B wasn't on anyone's radar.' It turned out a mutation in that unsuspected gene raises your risk for infection and tells whether the usual treatment at the time would work.

Researchers are exploring the entire genome of people affected in different ways by COVID-19. Patient outliers are of interest one type of outlier is severe cases that cannot be explained for example, someone who is under 50. The other outliers are people who have been exposed to the coronavirus again and again but, based on blood tests, never contract it. This suggests that they are intrinsically resistant to the infection itself. That it is possible for your genes to make you immune to an infectious disease.

Genes can make people immune to HIV norovirus and other illnesses that are passed from one person to another. Discoveries about the genetic roots of diseases should they arise could lead to improvements in prevention, diagnosis, and treatment. With information about who is most likely to get the disease, based on genes, health professionals could potentially offer tailored advice about prevention.

If a gene were to blame for sending otherwise healthy people to the intensive care unit, health providers could possibly observe certain COVID-19 patients with extra vigilance or provide extra preventive care after a positive test. When researchers discover a gene that can help or hinder a disease's progress, they can try to find or develop drugs that turn up or shut down that gene's activity.

It is not just a fever and coughing leading to shortness of breath, like everyone thought at first. Scientist discovered that this virus can be more than a respiratory disease, they call it 'great imitator' which makes it difficult to diagnose and even harder to treat. Because this is a new disease, virologist and epidemiological scientists are on the race against time to find a cure for this thing in the form of vaccine(s).

A new theory about the new coronavirus comes from a study in China. Researchers there were studying changes in coronavirus RNA over time to figure out how various coronaviruses are related to each other. They looked at 103 samples of new viruses from people and looked coronaviruses from animals. It turned out the coronaviruses found in humans were not the same, they were called L and S types. The S-type is the older strain, but the L-type was seen in the early stages of the outbreak and they suspect that one may cause more disease than the other. They are looking deeper at it.

Some reports have started to emerge about people who have recovered from COVID-19, three months later tested positive again. Several reports from China have described cases of people with mild symptoms continuing to test positive for the virus, even after recovery. A small study of Chinese healthcare workers also described findings where people continued to test positive even after they had recovered. The study found that these individuals no longer had symptoms and that they didn't go on to infect their family members.'

At this point Ntobs pauses momentarily, playing with a cursor of the laptop looking for an audio clip to share with her captivated audience. She finds the clip, before playing it, she takes a swig from a glass that has been sitting on table since she started talking. The glass has two lemon slices. To my mind, the pause provides a perfect moment to drop in a question or two. So, I take advantage of the opening giving myself permission to interrupt her presentation. This move turns to be a bad mistake.

'So, Ntobs what you are saying is that I should hold off popping the Champagne

because scientists are still a long way off making a breakthrough on a vaccine?' Next to me sits a doctor, an older gentleman who upon hearing me blowing my pipe appeared to frown a gesture betrayed by muscular twitching inside his horn-rimmed glasses, he shifts uncomfortably the moment I pop the question.

It seems there is a decorum governing the protocol around here. Unbeknown to me, my interjection reveals manners uncouth to the audience. The apparent breach undermines an unspoken rule holding the professionals gathered here today to a certain standard. By bursting out, I have appropriate to myself a right not given. A deeply flawed premise.

Aware that I am a newcomer to the INSIGHT FORUM, she chose not to make a big deal out of it, clearly my behaviour is out of kilter with the order here. Ntobs is magnanimous as she is diplomatic in handling the awkward moment. Before supplying an answer, she pauses to reflect.

'I guess in a way you could say that.' She immediately continues from there without waiting to see if there was a follow up on my initial question. 'Vaccines are coming soon but there is no silver bullet that will save the world from COVID-19.'

'Two cases outside of China are even more puzzling: people who had seemingly recovered and tested negative, then weeks later, began to have symptoms again and were found to be positive when re-tested. Research will continue to look at this question, but from what we know about our body's ability to fight of viruses, it is highly unlikely that a person that has recovered from COVID-19 and made antigen will become reinfected in such a short period of time.' She plays the clip. The video updates us on the current research in three facilities in USA, Germany, and China.

Vaccines work by training the immune system to recognise the virus before an infection occurs. Producing an effective vaccine will be a huge feather in the cap of the researchers, companies and nations involved both in terms of prestige of science and geopolitics. Since 1918 the Spanish flu virus is present today, we get the flu, but we do not die from it compared to the time of when it first broke out as the pandemic. After some months this will stop being an epidemic but become another virus, this we know for a fact based on our experiences of the previous outbreaks.

The coronavirus will not go away but it will not kill as much, it will be like a common cold where deaths still occur but in low numbers. All animals have viruses that live inside them. Bats, and several other mammal groups, are natural carriers of coronaviruses. These coronaviruses are not harmful to these animals but do pose a threat to humans if they jump between species, my research colleagues elsewhere have told us.

The coronavirus will certainly be present forever, but not as deadly as it was between January and December 2020. Then the pandemic phase will stop on its own. Some researchers have suggested that with lockdown, which in effect is reset button by doing as exactly what the quarantine protocol says we must do the world would need just three months and they should have been through it. Sadly, the world ignored this basic tool for fighting its spread instead, we are seeing a ferocious resurgence with catastrophic effect.

The University of Oxford scientists have launched phase I/III clinical trial of its vaccine made from a weakened version of a common cold virus, the adenovirus, taken from chimpanzees. The adenovirus is genetically altered so it is incapable of reproducing itself. The vaccine is combined with genes to trigger antibodies that allow the immune system to destroy the virus.

A flu shot, for example, contains the outer shell of the flu virus that your body's immune system learns to attack. This is what gives a person immunity. At the heart of every vaccine is an antigen – the thing which provokes the body to generate antibodies (proteins that stick to the antigen whenever they may find it) as immune responses. Antigens prevent virus particles from infecting other cells. Antigens are harvested from the blood of those infected. Many teams are looking at SARS-COV-2 vaccines that consist of a single protein mass produced by adding a gene for the protein that forms the outer coat to cell thereby produce the protein in a pure form.

The most novel of the vaccines to be produced in the future is aimed at genetic engineering called nucleic-acid vaccines or, mRNA vaccine. The vaccine uses something called the messenger RNA approach. This phase I trial started in mid-March. As of mid-April, three different doses were given to three groups of 45 healthy adults, ages 18 to 55. An additional six groups, with three groups of older adults ages 56 to 70 and three groups of adults ages 71 and above, had been added to this phase I study. Preliminary results were positive, says Colleen Hussey, a spokesperson for Moderna company.

This technology does not require a virus to make the vaccine. Scientists identified the sequence for a key protein on the surface of the SARS virus, called a spike protein. This protein is key for allowing the virus to enter cells when a person gets infected. The instructions for making that spike protein were encoded into an instruction molecule called mRNA.

When the vaccine containing the instruction molecule is injected, it travels to immune cells and triggers them to make copies of the spike protein as if the cells have been infected with the coronavirus. Other cells of the immune system then learn about the spike protein and can offer immunity if they encounter the coronavirus.

With an mRNA vaccine, rather than injecting fragments of the virus, this drug gives the body the genetic code it needs to produce lots of copies of these viral fragments. When the immune system sees the viral fragments, it learns how to attack them. An RNA vaccine essentially turns the body into its own vaccine manufacturing house.

The body's cell manufactures the antigen the vaccine produces for immune response. Nucleic-acid vaccines are independent of their viruses. DNA Vaccine: Phase I clinical trials have begun on a DNA vaccine from Inovio. The technology uses DNA designed to produce a specific immune response. A hand-held smart device that uses a brief electrical pulse to open small pores in the skin delivers the vaccine.

To build an mRNA vaccine, scientists only need access to the genetic sequence of SARS-nCov-2, and not the actual virus. They focus on the 'spike' protein which can then be used to synthesise an mRNA sequence, instructions that the cell can use to make the spike protein. The mRNA is then packaged in a lipid nanoparticle that serves as a delivery vehicle shuttling the instruction to our cell. Once inside the cells, the cellular machinery follows the mRNA instructions to produce the viral protein, which is then displayed on the surface of the cell and stimulates the immune system to mount a response.

The first coronavirus vaccine tested on humans has yielded positive results, with a small number of people who were tested showing an immunity against the virus. Moderna a pharmaceutical company based in Massachusetts said the vaccine called mRNA1273 was generally safe and well tolerated. The study has gone into phase 3 trial and expedited results are expected soon.

Pfizer and BioNTech were the second company to test four different variations of its mRNA vaccine on phase 3 trial, the first doses of the vaccine, called BNT162 were given to 360 people in Germany in May 2020. The researchers have since reported in November that the vaccine has 90% effectiveness. Following this trial, the company is now moving to produce thousands of millions of doses in 2021. The clip ends with background music I recognise it's a track from Nicky Minaj.'

Aware that she has been talking for some time, she paused yet again and asks her audience if she should continue another five minutes or so, as if they were on cue everybody replied in unison. 'We love this, please continue.'

'All the tests done during level 5 involve were taking a nasal swab and processing it in a Polymerase Chain Reaction (PCR) machine. There was an option of self-swab approach which was faster, protects health care workers from the risk of exposure, and should have let regulators approve swabbing in virtually any location instead of only at a medical centre. The PCR test is sensitive but expensive, it generally shows whether you have the virus even before you have symptoms or are infecting other people.

Another type of test being developed is called a Rapid Diagnostic Test (RDT). This would be like an in-home pregnancy test. Anyone can swab their nose the same way as for the PCR test, but instead of sending it into a processing lab, they would put it in a liquid container and then pour that liquid onto a strip of paper that would change colour if it detected the virus.

Even though it is not as sensitive as a PCR test, for someone who has symptoms it is quite accurate. You would still need to report your test result to your doctor, who would send it to the local clinic or coronavirus reporting forum.

Test turnaround times must result in identification of infected individuals within 24 hours. Isolation of infected individuals and contact quarantine must last for at least 14 days in designated community quarantine facilities. First and foremost, how many people have been infected and how many remain susceptible to this infection changes our view on the actual biology and pathogenicity of this virus. It will determine and change how we are looking at this virus.

Antibody tests also known as serology testing will also be essential for getting us out of our houses and back to work, and for easing the fear that has paralyzed the country. Policymakers will need to know how many people have the disease and how many have immunity against it before deciding when it's safe to loosen physical distancing requirements and when they will need to tighten up again to cope with the next wave of infections. Hopefully, having antibodies will protect someone from getting COVID- 19 a second time.

But since the virus has been detected only in November 2019, no one yet knows how long that protection will last. With the common cold a relative of the new coronavirus, immunity does not last long. You can catch it again a few months later. On the other hand, people who contracted severe acute respiratory syndrome in 2003 - 2004 still carry protective antibodies more than 15 years later.

If immunity lasts for years, those who have recovered can generally relax, resume their daily lives, and go back to hugging loved ones. If immunity lasts for just a short time, then even people who were infected once could be vulnerable again soon and it will be harder to develop a protective vaccine.

Researchers are also still deciding which antibodies their tests should look for. Some antibodies are made early in an infection and go away, usually within a few weeks, while others can linger for months or years. Looking for Immunoglobulin M, identify recent infections, while Immunoglobulin G, stays around longer. A third antibody, Immunoglobulin A, plays a role in the immune function of mucous membranes. Tests used for research also look for the number of antibodies. The amount is useful for a few reasons, including finding out if a person's blood is suitable for donating convalescent plasma.'

Making vaccine is a difficult process because it is both a political consideration and capital-intensive endeavour by the pharma industry players. Viral vaccinations are tricky because humans develop cell mediated immunity. Most vaccines that have been developed in the past 20 years have failed in clinical trials.

I cannot stress this enough, the complicating factor about this stuff is always the politics of access. Vaccines do not make financial sense to the pharma establishment because they benefit the low-income countries more, folks who do not have cash to buy these expensive drugs. This is counterintuitive if you think about. The question then arises, should the countries that finance the trials i.e. China, UK, Germany, USA, and Russia be the deciders?

Should the vaccine be first made available to the WHO the correct body via GAVI and Covax the funders' network so that it this body that decides where the crisis is the worst and make vaccine access there first. Should the vaccine be given to older people first and not young people? Shouldn't the global pharmacies share their IP with local pharmaceuticals to produce the vaccines? These are some of the questions that cannot be answered by scientists but by politicians.

I should like to add in the nature of things, governments and big business are clubs with closed membership. Expediency and self-serving national interests are the paramount factors in decisions-making process. Under such circumstances the question of equity get thrown out very quickly regardless of how altruistic their espoused intentions may be.

Vaccination is not going to offer humankind a viable exit from the straits that the COVID-19 pandemic has stuck it in. Here is why. COVID-19 vaccines, as far as I know will not 100 % prevent the disease but will provide a partial protection for a few months. A vaccine will not stop the virus, but it will protect people from dying from it.

This means that we may still catch the thing, but if we do, it will be in a much milder form that does not complicate our bodies. There will be a constant influx of few cases every day, usually ranging between asymptomatic and very mild, that usually do not require hospitalization, and which our local clinics should easily address without themselves being overwhelmed.

The last word is this, vaccines are not easy to make because viruses are complicated critters that mess up the immune system due to their ability to mutate often.

That a safe and effective vaccine will be found in 12 months is in my experience possible provided governments remove the red tape and can find ways to get it to people who need it most. This is doable.

Let us look at these statistics to make the point. We still have not got a vaccine for HIV, only a treatment regime. The search for a SARS vaccine has been ongoing since 2002 and has exhausted all available funding from governments. A vaccine for MERS has been sought since 2012 and nothing has been found yet despite efforts by the WHO and huge funding by the Saudi government. Both SARS and MERS are closely related to COVID-19. The first major outbreak of Ebola was in 2014 and the timeline there was 6 years, there have been developments to date, but more trials are needed before researchers can claim one.

The biggest issue with any vaccine is the safety considerations above everything else and testing for safety is a repeat exercise and that takes an awful lot of time. Researchers must satisfy themselves that whatever vaccine they produce will trigger an adaptive immune response in humans without showing toxicity. Plus, we must be satisfied that we understand the virus's characteristics and pathophysiology in humans.

We will live with coronavirus for months and years to come. Just about everyone is going to get infected with COVID-19 though the virus virulence will weaken with time. Some among us with bad health will die, some will get sick and recover all the same, others because of strong immune system will withstand the virus. It is an awfully slow process that will be sped up considerably with vaccinations. That is life.

When I say that COVID-19 is here to stay I do not mean that it is going to forever remain at pandemic level. Just for comparison, the Spanish flu was an H1N1 flu and remained with us for the whole century and still is without it being a pandemic.

What is going on right now is that in many parts of Asia COVID-19 has already started to slowly become endemic. Equally, it is important to state as a medical fact that coronavirus itself does not kill us per se. What happen is that it complicates the functioning of the body. Patients die from the resulting complications - the medical name of these complications is Cytokine and Bradykinesias storm. So, folks there is no need to panic we must learn to live with our new reality.

I have reviewed the marketing hype around the alcohol sanitiser. Most of the stuff that is out there does not meet the minimum standard of 70% alcohol content so, they do not protect the users. When you use hand sanitiser, it inactivates most of the viruses on your hands, the virus does not die or go anywhere. The good old Lifebuoy and Savlon bar soaps are good sanitisers because soap breaks the outer particle sticking on our skin and loosen the germs from your hands and the water washes it down the drain.

The idea of wearing gloves is a terrible one in a climate like South Africa. Also, keeping good distances between people when standing or seating in one place is going to be a regular thing to get used to from now on. No need to disinfect your home if there is no infected patient living in the house.

Tulio has already told us let us not worry too much about recovery treatment drugs instead advise our patients to eat for immunity. Tulio is right, here is another piece of advice. The lockdown measures worked to hobble the virus not to stop its spread. There is no social benefit in sheltering all humans from viral contact. Immunity is increased by exposure to pathogens not sitting isolated in your house, so the patients must get out as often as they can fearlessly, living life as it was meant to be lived –in all its messyness.

We have been living among viruses and other germs for aeons our immune system evolved in response to them. Little kids do not develop healthy immunity when their parents seal them off into Ziplock-bag. They get healthy by becoming exposed to the *gogatjies*.' The overhead projector goes blank and then the words, 'thank you for your time flash across and down its screen in multi-coloured finish. There is all round laughter and applause.

'I know I have delivered a lengthy talk and I am slow in my speech. I will now open Q&A session for the panel to address aspects not covered by Tulio or myself.'

Tulio rushes to the podium to make an administrative announcement wearing a big smile on his face no doubt pleased with Ntobs' performance. 'To my right, the panel is ready to deep-dive into the details of your questions. Please bear in mind, we are also joined by our online global audiences. As usual, the presentation material is available to our subscribers, if you are new to our forum – a reference to me no doubt - please send your details to Yvonne our Administrator to be included in our list. Light snack is served in the atrium outside the auditorium, please help yourselves.'

The Q&A session ended minutes before 6pm. A couple of guests left the building immediately, a few mingled at leisure while those without pressing work commitments continued informal discussion with the panellists.

※ ※

It has been twenty days since my last briefing. This morning, I am attending another session sponsored by Sanofi at their plush Sanofi House, Grand Central. The lead presenter is Dr. Nacinah, Head of Vaccines of the South African branch of the pharmaceutical giant. She opened her talk by saying, 'first, scientists discovered patients who had recovered from infection with coronavirus, but mysteriously didn't have any antibodies against it. Next it emerged that this might be the case for a significant number of people.

Then came the finding that many of those who do develop antibodies seem to lose them again after just a few months. In short, though antibodies have proved invaluable for tracking the spread of the pandemic, they might not have the leading role in immunity that we once thought. If we are going to acquire long-term protection, it looks increasingly like it might have to come from somewhere else.

But while the world has been preoccupied with antibodies, researchers have started to realise that there might be another form of immunity – one which, in some cases, has been lurking undetected in the body for years. An enigmatic type of white blood cell is gaining prominence. And though it has not previously featured heavily in the public consciousness, it may well prove to be crucial in our fight against COVID-19. This could be the T cell's big moment. When researchers tested blood samples taken years before the pandemic started, they found T cells which were specifically tailored to detect proteins on the surface of COVID-19.

T cells are a kind of immune cell, whose main purpose is to identify and kill infected cells. It does this using proteins on its surface, which can bind to proteins on the surface of these imposters. Each T cell is highly specific – there are trillions of possible versions of these surface proteins, which can each recognise a different target. Because T cells can hang around in the blood for years after an infection, they also contribute to the immune system's long-term memory and allow it to mount a faster and more effective response when it's exposed to an old foe.

Several studies have shown that people infected tend to have T cells that can target the virus, regardless of whether they have experienced symptoms. But scientists have also discovered that some people can test negative for antibodies against COVID-19 and positive for T cells that can identify the virus. This has led to suspicions that some level of immunity against the disease might be twice as common as was previously thought.

Most bizarrely of all, when researchers tested blood samples taken years before the pandemic started, they found T cells which were specifically tailored to detect proteins on the surface of COVID-19. This suggests that some people already had a pre-existing degree of resistance against the virus before it ever infected a human. And it appears to be surprisingly prevalent: 40% of unexposed individuals had these cells. It looks increasingly like T cells might be a secret source of immunity to COVID-19.

The central role of T cells could also help to explain some of the quirks that have so far eluded understanding – from the dramatic escalation in risk that people face from the virus as they get older, to the mysterious discovery that it can destroy the spleen.

Deciphering the importance of T cells is not just a matter of academic curiosity. If scientists know which aspects of the immune system are the most important, they can direct their efforts to make vaccines and treatments that work.

Most people probably have not thought about T cells, or T lymphocytes as they are also known, since school, but to see just how crucial they are for immunity, we can look to late-stage Aids. The persistent fevers. The sores. The fatigue. The weight loss. The rare cancers. The normally harmless microbes, such as the fungus Candida albicans – usually found on the skin – which start to take over the body.

Over the course of months or years, HIV enacts a kind of T cell genocide, in which it hunts them down, gets inside them and systematically makes them commit suicide. 'It wipes out a large fraction of them,' says Adrian Hayday, an immunology professor at King's College London and group leader at the Francis Crick Institute. 'And so that really emphasises how incredibly important these cells are – and that antibodies alone are not going to get you through.'

During a normal immune response to let us say, a flu virus – the first line of defence is the innate immune system, which involves white blood cells and chemical signals that raise the alarm. This initiates the production of antibodies, which kick in a few weeks later.

And in parallel with that, starting out about four or five days after infection, you begin to see T cells getting activated, and indications they are specifically recognising cells infected with the virus. These unlucky cells are then dispatched quickly and brutally – either directly by the T cells themselves, or by other parts of the immune system they recruit to do the unpleasant task for them – before the virus has a chance to turn them into factories that churn out more copies of itself.

Looking at COVID-19 patients – but also I'm happy to say, looking at individuals who have been infected but did not need hospitalisation – it's absolutely clear that there are T cell responses,' says Hayday. 'And almost certainly this is particularly good news for those who are interested in vaccines, because clearly we're capable of making antibodies and making T cells that see the virus. That's all good.'

In fact, one vaccine – developed by the University of Oxford – has already been shown to trigger the production of these cells, in addition to antibodies. It is still too early to know how protective the response will be, but one member of the research group told BBC News that the results were 'extremely promising.'

There is a catch, however. In many patients who are hospitalised with more serious COVID-19, the T cell response has not quite gone to plan. Vast numbers of T cells are being affected,' says Hayday. 'And what is happening to them is a bit like a wedding party or a stag night gone wrong – I mean massive amounts of activity and proliferation, but the cells are also just disappearing from the blood.' One theory is that these T cells are just being redirected to where they are needed most, such as the lungs. But his team suspects that a lot of them are dying instead.

Autopsies of COVID-19 patients are beginning to reveal what we call necrosis, which is a sort of rotting. This is particularly evident in the areas of the spleen and lymph glands where T cells normally live. Spleen necrosis is a hallmark of T cell disease, in which the immune cells themselves are attacked. T cells can lurk in the body for years after an infection is cleared, providing the immune system with a long-term memory. Dwindling T cells might also be to blame for why the elderly are much more severely affected by COVID-19.

Hayday points to an experiment conducted in 2011, which involved exposing mice to a version of the virus that causes Sars. Previous research had shown that the virus – which is also a coronavirus and a close relative of COVID-19 triggered the production of T cells, which were responsible for clearing the infection.

The follow-up study produced similar results, but the twist was that this time the mice could grow old. As they did so, their T cell responses became significantly weaker. However, in the same experiment, the scientists also exposed mice to a flu virus. And in contrast to those infected with COVID-19, these mice managed to hold onto their T cells that acted against influenza well into their twilight years.

It is an attractive observation, in the sense that it could explain why older individuals are more susceptible to COVID-19. When you reach your 30s, you begin to really shrink your thymus [a gland located behind your sternum and between your lungs, which plays an important role in the development of immune cells] and your daily production of T cells is massively diminished.

The fact that coronaviruses can lead to lasting T cells is what recently inspired scientists to check old blood samples taken from people between 2015 and 2018, to see if they would contain any that can recognise COVID-19. The fact that this was indeed the case has led to suggestions that their immune systems learnt to recognise it after being encountering cold viruses with the similar surface proteins in the past. While antibodies are still important for tracking the spread of COVID-19, they might not save us in the end.

If old exposures to cold viruses really are leading to milder cases of COVID-19, however, this bodes well for the development of a vaccine – since it is proof that lingering T cells can provide significant protection, even years after they were made. But even if this is not what is happening, the involvement of T cells could still be beneficial – and the more we understand what is going on, the better.

Vaccines if developed properly, provide an opportunity to induce the type of trained immunity that is optimal for mounting protective immune response, not only against this coronavirus but also against future pandemics.

The way vaccines are designed generally depends on the kind of immune response scientists are hoping to elicit. Some might trigger the production of antibodies – free-floating proteins which can bind to invading pathogens, and either neutralise them or tag them for another part of the immune system to deal with. Others might aim to get T cells involved, or perhaps provoke a response from other parts of the immune system.

The virus is evidently highly visible to the immune system, even in those who are severely affected. So, if we can stop whatever it is doing to the T cells of the patients, we have had the privilege to work with, then we will be a lot further along in controlling the disease. It seems likely that we are going to be hearing a lot more about T cells in the future. She concludes her talk.

※ ※

The presentation government made to MPs gives insight into the healthcare system's state of readiness: South Africa has just over 60 million people, and it expected 2million of its citizens to be infected. According to this presentation the country has less than half the number of ventilators needed to deal with peak infection. Government hospitals has 1 111 working ventilators, with 2 105 in the private hospitals for a total of 3 216 ventilators. According to projections the healthcare system would need 7 000 ventilators to deal with the virus, a shortage of 3 784. Denel was asked to make the shortfall.

There are currently only 3 318 critical care beds available, with 2 140 of those in private hospitals; there are 2 722 high care beds in the country, with only 1 082 of those in the government hospitals; there is a total of 119 416 hospital beds available, across South Africa. Politics could still see some people trampled underfoot in the rush to get out.

During peak infection in an optimistic scenario, and with one lockdown enforced, the peak need for beds in intensive care units could exceed 14 700 beds at the highest level, and 4 100 in the lowest level. The presentation said that, only severe Covid-19 patients will be treated at hospitals, while moderately infected patients will be accommodated at field tents where only the basic medical care will be provided.

But we all know, and government acknowledges it, that testing is inadequate and needs to be expanded. Targeted testing of high-risk groups, returning travellers, those in contact with infected patients would have enabled the government to quarantine infected persons earlier. Who is tested, was more important than how many tested? Testing was significant for another reason, it was likely to throw up a higher positive rate of diagnosis, all other things being equal.

The more you test, the lower the positive diagnosis rate. Importantly, South Africa shows a lowering rate too. That means we would have been a country with a low rate of testing and a low positive diagnosis rate, probably not a good position to be at for herd immunity. A good example is Japan, which had a low rate of testing, a low positive diagnosis rate, a low number of cases per million and low mortality.

We were inundated with fake news on social media platforms, incomplete information from the official channels and information overload from news media. Questions around self-isolation versus mandatory quarantine, getting tested when fitting case definition versus asking for the test after exposure from known infected person. Generic OTC medicine versus sleeping the virus out. PCR testing kit for the presence of the virus versus rapid antigen testing kit for presence of antibodies remained in a state of flux.

※ ※

The South African Covid-19 Modelling Consortium is a group of researchers from academic, government institutions and non-government organisations. Developing a multidisciplinary process, a mathematical model to simulate the spread of a disease in the context of public health. The group included epidemiologists, virologists, actuaries, intensivists, clinicians, and demographers. The group used the National Covid Epi Model software. This model generated the projections, comprised a set of formal assumptions about how the world might work.

WHO recommends test positivity rate should not be allowed to exceed 10% at most, with 5% or lower being the goal? Any more than the higher level and you are not doing anywhere near enough and should be locking down rapidly, because the disease is already out of control. To say any increase is not due to increased testing you should remain below the lower value. Above the higher threshold and you are being bombed to smithereens, unless you are below the lower number any increase is certainly real and probably undercounted.

These experts have given input based on their own experience and on their knowledge of the global literature to inform the values used in the models. The current version of the model estimated that South Africa can expect total of 12 million symptomatic cases of COVID-19 to have accumulated by early November 2020. The epidemic would peak around 1 million active cases in late August. Overall, they estimated that 88% of the population would be infected, most would have mild symptoms or none. About 1% was expected to develop severe symptoms sick enough to require hospitalisation.

When looking at long term projections the group gave two possible scenarios, optimistic and pessimistic. Under optimistic scenario they assumed that the level 5 lockdown reduced the contact rate by 60%, the level 4 reduced the contact rate by 35% and level 3 by 20%. Under the pessimistic scenario, they assumed that the level 5 reduced contact rate by 40% level 4 by 25% and level 3 by 10%.

South African does not and could not know the true number of people infected with COVID-19. The number of laboratory-confirmed cases depended on the testing criteria and testing capacity of the labs. Therefore, the true number of people infected with COVID-19 is much higher than the number of cases reported publicly.

Based on this projection, the group expected hospital capacity to be overwhelmed, with all ICU beds in both public and private sector filled up by July. The group made a caveat that this was dependent on individual behaviour change and tighter or looser restriction regime. Since the proportion of infected individuals who remained asymptomatic, and the relative infectiousness and the duration of infectiousness of these asymptomatic individuals give rise to uncertainty. This has implications for the transmission dynamics in the model and the projected number of hospitalisations and deaths.

The said, 'we can each of us help continue to flatten the curve by reducing our contacts, observing physical distancing, washing our hands often, wearing non-medical masks, isolating ourselves when we are sick and quarantining when we have been in contact with someone who was infected. Changing the course of the epidemic is our shared responsibility.'

The benefit of the behaviour change is to reduce the infection rate dramatically so that, instead of doubling every eight days, it goes down every eight days. Exponential growth is not intuitive because R0 is hard to measure. If you say that 2 percent of the population is infected and this will double every eight days, most people will not know that in 40 days, many of the township folks will be infected.

We use the reproduction rate to calculate how many new infections are caused by an earlier infection. We know it is below R1 wherever the number of infection cases is going down and above +R1 wherever the number of cases is going up. If you started with 100 infections in Thembisa, after 40 days you would end up with 17 infections at the lower end of R number and 3,200 at the higher end of the R number. The active flattening only occurs when R is maintained below 1 through public health measures.

If we dismiss the rather disturbing implications of failed testing and tracing strategy in much of the country and take the disease trajectory as it is, we need to ask whether an R of 1.2 represents a concern. To the government it does not. However, if we project the trajectory forward at the current level of R, we can expect exponential new infections where the numbers become seriously out of control. The failure to test and trace adequately at scale is distorting our understanding of the trajectory.

By the middle of May South Africa was the only Afrikan country with the highest rate of infections and growing in the continent. Western Cape and Gauteng were the provinces with the most recorded cases of infections. In my province, the city of Joburg city followed by Kempton Park had the most confirmed numbers. SA's COVID-19 trajectory was unique because unlike most other countries, although it did not follow an exponential increase in cases in its first 100 days this changed midway through July. In statistical terms, the earlier picture showed a case recovery rate of 18.05% as per data.

Funeral gatherings were going on despite their proven risk for spreading community transmissions. Social grants pay points and food distribution points people pilling on top of one another. Vulnerable old people instead of being shielded had to stand in long queues without physical distancing for hours on end.

The combination of excessive law enforcement and non-essential measures together with the failure to take forward common sense measures has given rise to losing trust of communities. The containment of imported cases primarily among flying travellers and tourists, served to arrest the spread but did not flattened the curve as the government had initially purported to do.

We know that in Vo an Italian town 3,300 people were tested twice, of those who were found to be infected 50-75% had no symptoms at the time of the test and never developed symptoms. A 20-year-old Chinese woman had infected five relatives with the virus even though she never displayed any symptoms herself. Apparently healthy people could be unknowingly spreading the virus. In short, the government was in a better position to lead a data-driven response based on the spread or absence of the virus.

Containment and mitigation tend to happen on a geographic basis attacking the hotspot at the source. Quarantine remained our best hope in responding to the outbreak. High-density communities like in the people living in the shack community could not socially distance and therefore did not benefit from the lockdown. The talk about the 'highest or lowest' number of infections in a country is a false narrative. In truth, we expect many people in the world to be infected with the virus.

On the other hand, mitigation started with the idea that we will probably not drive transmission to zero, so then we start thinking about what we can do to prepare our hospitals and communities to reduce transmissions. In the period of lockdown, government set up field hospitals, imported ventilators and bought personal protective clothing for the frontline workers.

When an area meets the gating criteria, it enters a phase according to which vulnerable groups should continue to shelter in place and maximise physical distance from others including avoiding social settings of more than 50 people as the precautionary measures.

Specific types of formations, which included churches under this phase were regulated to operate under strict physical distancing protocols. The rules defining strict, moderate, and limited physical distancing protocols kept changing depending on who was speaking, however.

It is hard to think of any policy ever having been imposed so widely with such little preparations. The closing down of society was not a thought-out response, so much as a desperate measure for a desperate time. In other parts of the world, governments were successful in slowing down the pandemic the opposite was true for South Africa. The needless shutdown was taken at a high cost to the economy and the livelihoods of millions of South Africans.

I suddenly remembered that the idea of a lockdown was to slow down the rate of infection so that the infection is spread evenly out over time, in order that fewer people are sick at any one time so that hospitals have the sufficient capacity to attend to the very sick and give them a chance to recover. What this meant was that the same number of people will still get infected, just not all at the same time. That is what flattening the curve means. Maybe the government objectives changed midway we were not made aware.

To prevent infections at all testing and contact tracing (trace, test and treat) was the best first response in the suite of strategies available. Containment strategy is used at the start of an outbreak. It involves tacking the spread of a disease within a community, and then using individual quarantine to keep people who have been infected from spreading it. The reason that we want to find those people early is so that we can make sure that they stay out of circulation in the community and also that they get the care that they need as soon as they need it.

The question was whether the lockdown period was used properly by the government? The required protocols for employers, schools and public health authorities should also have been developed, tested, and deployed. The NHLS capacity to test was around 19,500 a day in August, a number too low to manage the scale needed post lockdown. Also, South African buys most of its PPEs from outside the country a factor that slows down the work of nurses and doctors because many refused to work without the protective clothing those who braved it died in the line of duty.

20 infected people would likely require public health authorities to trace the contacts from forty to a hundred people per week, with a better than 80% success rate. Contact tracing is time-intensive work. It would take about a hundred person-hours of work to trace the contacts of each confirmed case of the COVID-19. But if done quickly, and at the proper scale, the method can be effective. How we behave in response to the pandemic determined whether we were successful in reducing the spread of the infection in and around our communities.

Was it reasonable for people to ask whether the behaviour change was necessary? The answer is yes. There might be a few areas where the number of cases would never have gotten large numbers of infections and deaths, but there was no way to know in advance which areas those would be. Stay-at-home measures work because when everyone decides to stay home, everyone's decisions affect everything. The change allowed us to avoid many millions of deaths and extreme overload of the hospitals, which would also have increased deaths from other causes what is known as 'excess' death.

That is why, even now, we listen with rapt attention to the news cycle as scientists explain to us the way that the virus spreads and the ways that we can minimise it. Certainly, this disease has taught us that it is not just my decisions that matter.

Shutdowns were understandable and defensible in the beginning, when we did not entirely know what we were up against. Later as more information became available, we became less jittery and more stable. Now we need a more moderate response, one that let us fix the issues the shutdown created while still allowing us to keep a lid on the worst of the virus.

SARS-nCoV-2 is not a computer model. It is communicated by humans in conditions conducive to transmission. If community transmission is not interrupted through change in human behaviour and prevention programmes, it spreads and indeed it did that.

The national consensus that was there initially started to fray when it became increasingly difficult to understand the behaviour of the ministers unable to explain the rationale behind government decisions. Regulations were enacted without explaining what the supporting evidence was and what scientific advice was given to guide us. The nation increased its disillusion. You should remember that government suffers under poor leadership and deteriorating governance in general, but more so under climate of incompetence. We were extra vigilant against government excesses.

※ ※

Tonight, the president stands ready behind the lectern at the GCIS auditorium about to commence yet another address to the nation. The third in five weeks. He is re-emphasising the message, 'stay at home and wear a face covering' the government's consistent messaging and also the means by which the easing of the lockdown from level 5 to 4 can be made possible. Four may be five minutes into his speech the president is eager to show his audience the correct use of a face mask. He dives straight to the nub of matter.

Using his left hand, he grabs *isfonyo*, anxious to keep his eyes on the tele-prompter, he picks up the cloth lying beside the mic on the lectern. He fumbles putting the cloth in place. He tries placing the cloth with his right hand the second time and when that too fail, he abandoned the attempt leaving the face mask stuck on his face rather clumsily. I know many felt sorry for the president in his moment of embarrassment at the wardrobe malfunction. I did not share this sentiment.

I am thinking that this is reminiscent of the days of Zuma comedies only marginal improvement. In his nine-year stint Zuma, the avuncular grandpa, was a downright jack providing the same level of entertainment as Joni the Trump. I remember this one moment when he could not get the word 'deterioration' rolling off his tongue. I have nothing but the most respect for this Nkandla crooner for his boldness.

Mr. President do not ever do this to yourself again if you have not tried it at home first with your kids, please do not try it when the cameras have started rolling. It is considered bad manners to fumble a simple task like putting on a face cloth on your face, it shows just how much you treat your audience watching on public television with total disdain. If you are going to be this daring at least ask for their permission and their forgiveness in advance.

The president had a choice to interrupt his address for few seconds, grab the cloth with both hands making sure it is in place as correctly as he wanted to show it then proceed with his speech. How difficult can that be? How is it even possible to empathise with an elementary error like that. Mr president, I was wrong to think you were smarter than Zuma. Next time, to avoid looking like an imbecile in front of a worried nation, I implore you rehearse your speech and the theatre that goes with it before you appear live on-camera. You have 300 people working for you in the presidency they would be more than willing to give a helping hand. President, you can thank me later for this sage advice.

At some point, I must leave home and venture into public spaces. The new rules are different and confusing. In public places I am required to wear a cloth face covering and do physical distancing. Inside the store, I must stand two arm's length apart from the next shopper. There are persplex barriers hanging between me and the cashier that act as a form of protection from me. Everything points to me as the carrier of the disease knowing it or not. Can this presumption be correct, I doubt it?

A few months back anyone wearing a face mask in public would have drawn freak stares and funny comments from those watching from a distance. Now a face mask is reminder of the strange times we live in.

If it was not hilarious I wouldn't have had to laugh, I could not help but notice folks in long queues at Sangweni Plaza some wearing homemade cut-outs from pantyhose, kitchen towels, bra pads, denim cloths with lots of gaps in between the nose and mouth. The parts of the face to protect most fiercely are the nose and eyes.

Some opted for a scarf wrapped round their face, others make do with a T-shirt yanked up over their mouth. The more creative hook colourful homemade varieties around their ears, while the lucky few wear distinctive medical grade N95 respirators. Facemasks like handwashing are cheap and do not impose hidden costs.

To be sure, wearing face masks is utterly useless in preventing the COVID-19 because if sneezed at by an infected carrier the virus is small enough to penetrate through the filter is made of it can infect the person standing opposite that individual. That said, one of the reasons widespread public face masks wearing is important has to do with the prevalence of asymptomatic carriers who can still spread virus to others without them knowing it.

Face masks are a symbol of the pandemic era - a visual metaphor for this unseen foe. If everybody is wearing a face mask, that would mean infected and asymptomatic people are also wearing masks we are protecting one another. This could help reduce the amount of virus which gets into the environment. Face masks and their problem with breathing and bad breadth accumulating on the mouthpiece and making it harder to recognise facial expressions of those we talk to is the trade-off we make for our freedom to walk the streets.

One study showed that we spray thousands of droplets invincible to the eye into the air just by uttering the words 'stay healthy.' A single cough can spread up to 3000 droplets in four to six metres distances. Another study found that the virus was remarkably resilient in aerosol form compared with other forms of viruses. If combined with physical distancing, face masks are useful in reducing transmission in the community particularly in gathered setting like taxis, buses and crowded indoor shops.

The best cloth face masks use at least 2 layers of a tightly woven cotton fabric but the one I liked best is a mask layered with a coffee filter inside. A cotton bandana is the worst covering you can wear, followed by a woollen scarf. A 600-thread-count pillowcase could filter out around 60% of the viral particles.

The most effective ones used multiple fabric layers such as silk, cotton flannel, felted wool, quilting cotton, and polyester materials were found to be effective. The problem with face cloth mask is right there, they are not meant to protect the wearer they leave other vulnerable parts of the face exposed, like the eyes. They are meant to keep an asymptomatic person from spreading it to others. If the 'other' is not wearing any covering that becomes a nuisance.

At a subsequent INSIGHT FORUM presentation, Tulio had disagreed with the face mask following recent findings from various studies. He told us, 'it is better to talk about face shields instead. Some doctors say it is time to take protection a step further and try full face shields as restrictions slowly begin to loosen.

Face shields are nothing new in medical settings doctors and nurses who treat coronavirus patients are using them along with standard face masks. Face shields together with physical distance of two metres or more appear to have several benefits from community transmission: They are easy to wear correctly and good at blocking droplets, they are really a better option for protection. Wearing face shields may help prevent the spread of COVID-19 by protecting the wearer from droplets carrying the virus.

Perencevich and his colleagues published a report in *JAMA* in May, arguing that face shields have more COVID-fighting potential than standard masks when used with increased testing, contact tracing, and physical distancing. A few things make shields superior he says. For one, many people wear masks that do not fit well, so they do not work as well. They also prompt people to touch their faces more, increasing the risk of viral spread. They leave much to be desired in terms of comfort, he says, and they make it harder to breathe.

Shields come with the perk of being easily sanitized and reused. Unlike masks, clear shields also allow for better communication people can read facial expressions, and those who are hearing impaired can read lips, he says. Shields have been found to successfully block droplets. One cough simulation study found that a shield may reduce exposure by 96 % when worn within 18 inches of someone coughing.

'School children in Singapore and Korea are being given face shields as they headed back to classes. I think it would be cool if not funky to wear one, especially if you're sick or immunocompromised.' Tulio told his gathered audience at one of his briefings. He was suitably impressed.

※ ※

In the fog of pandemic, every statistic tells a story, but no one statistic tells the whole story. The explanations for the case-death gap were complementary, rather than competing theories in the coronavirus story. Deaths lag cases —that explain something, but it does not explain everything. You cannot have a serious discussion about case and death numbers without noting that people die of diseases after they get sick. It follows that there should be a lag between a surge in cases and a surge in deaths.

More subtly, there can also be a lag between the date a person dies and the date the death certificate is issued. The death lag is probably the most important thing to understand in evaluating the case-death gap. Even where deaths are rising, corresponding cases are rising notably faster.

In early months of 2020, the novelty of the coronavirus meant that doctors had no idea what to expect. Health-care professionals were initially shocked that what they assumed to be a respiratory disease was causing blood clots, microvascular thrombosis, and organ damage. But millions of cases and hundreds of white papers later, we know more. That is how, for example, doctors know the prescription of the steroid dexamethasone to rein in out-of-control immune responses that destroy patients' organs is helpful in the overall management of cases. Mortality declined in Italian and British hospitals when they were not overrun with patients. This is another reason why flattening the curve is not just a buzzy slogan, but a matter of life and death. As hospitals across the nation started to fill up, we saw hospital mortality increases again.

The transition to summer may have stamped out other illnesses that were weakening our immune systems. People in the Northern Hemisphere may absorb more Vitamin D in the summer, which might mitigate COVID-19 mortality. As would be witnessed later in the year in some parts of Europe the virus had a variance that became more contagious, but not more deadly, which might — in combination with other factors, like superior hospital treatment of the disease — exacerbate an outbreak in cases that doesn't correspond with an increase in deaths.

Finally, as more people wear masks and move their activities outside in the summer, they might encounter smaller infecting doses of COVID-19. Some epidemiologists have claimed that there is a relationship between viral load and severity. With more masks and more outdoor interactions, it is possible that the recent surge is partly buoyed by an increase in these low-dosage cases.

The case-death gap remains a bonfire of unknowns. And, as we have seen, uncertainty is a cavity where propaganda can breed. So, let us conclude with what we know for sure: The surge in cases represents a tragic failure — even if it does not lead to a correspondingly dramatic spike in deaths. This virus is a cryptic devil. It can brutalize people's bodies for weeks or months, even if it does not kill them.

It can savage the lungs of young people, even when it does not produce other symptoms. Those who are infected can transmit it to more vulnerable people. Those who contract severe cases can be sent to the hospital for weeks and live for months — which may turn into years — with aftershocks from the illness. Outbreaks might make school openings implausible, sports improbable, and ordinary life impossible.

The summer surge is an exceptional failure, born of weak leadership and terrible public-health communication. After all the graphs, statistics, science, and interpretations, we are left with a simple fact: thousands of South Africans died every day of a disease they could have avoided just by avoiding gathered masses and staying at home. If that's success, I pray I never live long enough to see what failure look like.

※ ※

When rumours of resurgence swirled panic among the world leaders was palpable. Not so with the infectious diseases experts. The rumours were not a concern for the scientists because they knew the facts and saw the evidence that emerged ahead of the curve. And so, it did not come as a surprise that the resurgence was happening, virologists and epidemiologists predicted it and when trends began to pattern out on their radar screens they knew it and were prepared to deal with the eventualities.

Many European countries saw cases ticking up sharply, triggered by premature relaxation of control measures, and public fatigue with face masks and distancing. Governments were at crossroads either impose harsher lockdown measures with stiffer penalties or letting the virus run its course. There was no middle ground. Most chose the former route without much success.

Experts worry that early success may have given many countries a false sense of security. The resurgence is a warning sign, says Ben Cowling, an epidemiologist at the University of Hong Kong. Many people, and even some in the scientific community, thought handling the crisis would be like a hurricane lockdown, where once it is gone, life can go back to normal, he says. With COVID-19, that is not what is going to happen. Leaders who embraced prompt and transparent evidence-based communication of risk, cost, and benefit to the citizenry including the measures that contain the outbreak had better success rate. The Asian nations is the case in point.

Even countries that so far had a stellar pandemic report card must keep working to fine-tune their messaging and sustain public support for control measures. Changing directives for instance on masks, can lead to more pushback in some places, especially among those in their 20s where anti-restriction sentiment is voiced the strongest.

Towards the end of October, the coronavirus entered a second wave in major jurisdictions no less ferocious, dynamic, and widespread in its tracks. Countries that had previously successfully contained the first wave for five months or more began experiencing the resurgence.

France and Germany were the first European countries to go back to hard national lockdown just five months after the previous lockdown. Many countries soon followed. The U.K. endured a painful third wave, far worse than its European neighbours like Spain, France, Italy and Germany. Then four weeks later, the Genome platforms reported that there was a variation to the existing viral strain with high infectivity upping the ante.

This virus evolves at a rate of one substation every 11 days. More people got infected at speed not previously seen. Steven Goldstein, an evolutionary virologist said, 'every variant wants to be more transmissible so the fact that so many of them are landing on these mutations suggest there could be a real benefit for the virus.' These different lineages are essentially arriving at the solution for it to interact more efficiently with human receptor ACE2. There is N601Y, a mutation that occurs in all three variants of the UK, RSA and Brazil, which replaces the coronavirus's 501st amino acid asparagine with tyrosine. This pattern is what scientists refer to as convergent evolution and is a sign of more trouble coming our way. This new development was like a cat among pigeons. Questions over the efficacy of the vaccines that were already given emergency approval for immunization will now intensify.

Saturday 13th May
Skin hunger

The sun slink below the skyline, forming a wavering backdrop to the building. Chichi put a hand on his cheek. His face felt as hot to the touch as Adebayo had, and his ebony skin had begun to take on a pinch, a wrinkled appearance that indicated dehydration. Chichi looked at him ponderously and up close without turning his face. Ade squirmed under Chichi's scrutiny, feeling as though his cousin was reading his thoughts. His symptoms came suddenly but took a long time to leave. The stay at home and put on face masks advice came a tad too late for Ade.

Saturday, May 13th Ade 28, remembers exactly. One day he felt perfectly fine and the next he was hit with a fever and severe body aches including headache and fatigue that was unremitting. Currently, there are only a few hundred confirmed cases of COVID-19 and maybe under ten deaths in Kempton Park. By May 18th, his condition had worsened noticeably. 'The fatigue was intense, and the coughing was frequent and dry, 'I felt like I was choking, like someone was grabbing me by my throat.' He says. Chichi is right Ade needs to go to hospital. But no one takes the first step.

The cock-a-doodle-doo of a rooster edged out a nonsensical dream, I stretched and rubbed my eyes as a lemony slice of sunshine pierced through the window. Soft taffeta-like sounds and muffled scurrying sounds filled me with helpless dread. I went to check on Ade. His fever had become worse overnight. A knife of guilt punctured me as I felt I probably should have checked on him during the night.

'Yo, Dude, you are going to fuckin die, you know.'

'You don't get to die here I am taking you to the freaking hospital. Come on, put on your fuckin clothes. Here wear this'

'Let us go, like now, okay.'

It took all my strength and Chich's getting Ade into the backseat of the car, a lime green Land Rover Vogue. He walked erratically, as if his right leg was shorter than his left leg. He reminded me of a car stuck in a sand bed. Chichi and I settled Ade between a pillow and blanket to support him on both sides. Nothing is more deadly than a deserted, waiting street. The trees were still; the mockingbirds were silent. The carpenters next door to our apartment had parked their tools for the day.

Chichi climbed inside and buckled down his seatbelt. He pulled forward and navigated the SUV onto a narrow but rock-strewn street and drove away. Ade sat up straight and adjusted the pillow, then in a slow motion rubbed his eyes as though to wipe the ordeal away. His vitality seemed to have evaporated as quickly as the brief morning rain. 'God go with you Bro.' Said Azu to a car that had long disappeared around the bend.

    As the Rover sped past by the boys perched atop the burlap cartons whooped and waved at us. Chichi waved back. Beyond the veld several men unloading cider block and sacks of cement from a truck, a fine powder of cement dust turned their faces ashy like a statue in a forgotten mine. They laughed and joked as they worked, seeming to enjoy one another's company.

    On the outskirts of the town the landscape changed. The depression of verdant grasses and coarse bushes lay slightly lower than the land around it so that it had a secret view towards the horizon and the inky hump of hills. It was pretty. Then the suburbs in the distance. Here the between was stark and barren. Scruffy palm trees poked up occasionally amidst the rubble and rubbish that littered the veld. The earth is brown and without grass. Motorcycles hurtle past us, honking. Signboards slide past, cluttering the roadside. Most of them were once white and are now brown with mud from the previous rain.

    After two bad turns, Chichi finally turned onto Chareron Road and followed the signs, many of them painted on the sides of the new buildings. Hospital park is on our right. As he approached the main gate, every available space seemed taken by the informal business mushrooming alongside the pavement. Some vendors had just arrived preparing to set up their wares for the day. Chichi bounced through the NetCare Waterfall gates. The dust floats in through the open windows to settle on my skin and eyes.

    Several kiosks were no more than blankets spread on the sidewalk. In front of ramshackle sheds on the roadside, women are bent over smoky roasting basins, fanning corncobs. Some displayed their wares – plucked chickens heads, legs and liver, dried fish, and fruits and vanilla flavoured Magewu in plastic bottles. He squeezed the Vogue into a narrow space between a pothole and the gate of the main entrance 'Hang in there Nja'yam, ses' fikile.'

    Ade shrugs he says nothing. We take him out of the car walking slowly; his limp more noticeable, his body moving sideways with each step. We are close to the reception when he turns to me and says, 'Thank you, *nne*.' It is one of the few times in the past three hours that he has spoken without being first spoken to. I do not want to think about why he is thanking me. I only know that suddenly and instinctively, I smell the damp and acid like breath. His voice sounded nasal, as if he needed to blow his nose. His eyes are jaundiced, so yellow they look dyed. I reach out and place my arm under his shoulder and he leans on me as we lift him to the stretcher. He cracked a dim smile.

    The nurse puts his toothpick into his shirt and grabs the stretcher placing him on his back. He disappears behind the screening room. Then he leads Chichi and I to an airless room with benches on both sides of a low table. 'I will do the screening and the doctor will do the clinical assessment shortly.' We sit on the opposite ends of the table, touching fists. We wait without talking.

By the time Ade was moved to the dedicated coronavirus ward, a specially created marque adjacent to the main building, his blood pressure was low, heart rate was racing, chest X-ray showed partial pneumonia on the lungs. He was admitted and tested positive for SARS-CoV-2. The nurse told us.

Ade was put on oxygen therapy spending a total of five days in the isolation ward with three other male patients whom he could not see their faces. They were not only having trouble with breathing, but also struggling with the isolation itself. His symptoms improved. On the May 23$^{rd.}$ he was discharged. We came to fetch him home. As he left the hospital the dry cough became wet but persistent for three more weeks. He was coping despite the cough. Eventually, he regained strength.

Although the cough never left him for weeks after discharge, he nevertheless survived the ordeal thanks to his youth. Like Ade more than seventy million people have been on the road to recovery world-wide that had been infected. Over 80% of people did not have severe disease, most recovered in time and fully a few had lingering complaints of sorts, a handful had long Covid. When Ade took the second test, the virus could not be detected. A good result. Doctors cleared him to socially mix again.

Because Ayobami inserted me in the middle of the brothers, they reluctantly embrace me as one of their own. Even so, I shall remain the black sheep of the clan, I trust we are capable of caring and being considerate and be more tolerable human beings. I decide to keep an unobtrusively presence observing the goings-on off centre.

Adebayo, Chimamanda and Azuka maintained to anyone who cared to listen that they are cousins. Three brothers from different provinces of Nigeria. I remain unsure how each is related to the other. What makes me nervous is I am their fourth non-Nigerian brother living in the same commune.

Ade is from Lagos. He is gawky. He recently started working as a bartender at the Orange Hotel, a lodging outfit on the eastern part of Kempton Park two years ago. He was employed to bus tables, but after few incidents the manager thought it wise to move him to the dispatch where there were fewer valuable things to break.

Although his gravelly laughter made others in the dispatch direct their jokes towards him, he still regarded himself a stand-up comedian, the point around which laughs revolves. The dispatch crew made a proper contest of it. To see him from across the street, the serious young lad heaving his freight of the world's knowledge was to witness a scene that might have been a scene illustrated by an accomplished novelist.

Ade can squeeze water from dry rocks. His concept of making jokes is strangely funny. It is not the content of the material he uses to fire up others, it is him that is the social study of 'funny.' Self-deprecation is his signature tool. As soon as people gather around him wave of laughter crests through, a rogue swell of guffawing and rippling fits of lung-hacking hahas riptide the audience. Ade once told his colleagues the following, which I did not find funny.

> There are certain colours that you know will fade
> Almost immediately after purchasing
> A crimson lake about to drown itself in dirty brown
> A sky blue, cloudy with a chance of looking like shit
> An ochre, sandwiched between black and peach
> It is like you can see a future filled with disappointment
> Wrapping itself around the optimism of a pair of bright sandals.'
> Tapfunwa wears Cayambe navy multis. He wants to suck the juice out of life.
> He knows the world eats idealists, but damn…
> He says there is something beautiful about the gap between expectation and reality. Tapfunwa is a shitty boyfriend. Like, do you really wanna bleed for these stacks?
> Shelves and shelves, John would fuck me!
> Or, at least, he would not categorically scorn me.
> The only thing worse than categorical scorn is continuous scorn.
> That is a data joke. But seriously.
> The only thing worse than categorical scorn is imperative scorn.
> That is a serious joke, but badly done.

Chimamanda prefers the hipster version of his name, Chichi. He is still in his pyjamas and his black hair has a significant amount of salt and pepper for someone who has not yet crossed thirty. It makes him look dignified, particularly when he wears glasses, which he often does. He is tall and lanky all his T-shirts appear too small when he stretches. This guy never works out. He has a monthly membership at Planet Fitness at Glen Marais I think he has used it maybe twice in two and half years.

He is naturally lean and runs sometimes on Saturdays if he woke up early. He is so buttoned-up most of the time you would not think he is a great flirt. He has a great witty mind. It is one of the things his cousins love most about him. Chichi's gift among us is to weave realism out of extremity. He plants his flag where the ordinary and the astonishing meet where everyday people pause to wonder how exactly it came to this.

Azu has a habit of keeping his earmuffs permanently blocking out noises even when he is not listening to house music. This is his way of keeping a distance between himself and the rest of us. A boundary of some kind. An insurance against accidental chatting he otherwise would prefer not to entertain. Conversations lately have tended to be one sided with little or nothing to engage him. Perhaps it is that Azu has constructed a fantasy for his temporary habitation. He offers himself escape, but the kind that depends on and is inseparable from the world beyond. Escape that offers boundaries between himself and the rest of the world. Us in the room.

Azu is the opposite of Chichi in all things. Chichi is thin, Azu large. Chichi does not drink Azu drinks like fish. Chichi is a suit man, Azu lives all his life in graffiti decorated T-shirts and super low-cut jeans hanging loose on his butt. Azu is a fearless, outspoken artist and Chichi a self-conscious, introverted teacher. He was a rebellious teenager, Chichi tried to be the good boy, at least until he moved out of his parent's house at 18. Chichi has a degree in economics, Azu an aspiring photographer whose studio is a labyrinth of lights and darkness in the unused granny's flat at the back.

Ade is back from hospital a week now. The brothers want to take the boredom out of the house Azu and Chichi conjured up an idea they would like to keep hush hush for now until it comes to fruition. A party with a difference. Both are agreed that featuring important, successful people including high-profile lawyers, politicians, doctors and journalists and beautiful girls will be an excellent idea to boost their profiles. However, they got stuck at drawing a guest list. In Chichi's list, artists and Rastafarians that are permanent feature of Azu circle of friends are not included. That is a problem for Azu.

Azu reminiscence of a party he organised in December for his girlfriend, Mando. The gig was an over-subscribed event by members of the local chapter of the Rastafarian commune. It was dope. The gig went on until the booze from the supplying tavern was stocked out. The cops were forced to intervene on two occasions, once to attend to reports of fights that had broken out between a Rasta man and a random guy who strayed into the party. The next time to shut party the down because according to the commander in charge of the responder unit was 'gatvol with their shit' he told Azu.

On the other hand, earlier in March before the lockdown, Chichi had attended an 'Oyster' party at a house owned by a child of a minister where the guests turned up bearing Merlot, Malbec, Glenlivet, Whisky and expensive Russian Vodka in their hands. Men in good moods and just-so trainers, women with varying degrees of miniskirts and fake hare, their curls, their tresses, their long straight manes trailing down their backs as they walked into music, like so many Beyoncé's. To Chichi's mind, this is the kind of party he wanted to host.

Chichi is motivated not to miss another opportunity. Previously, at that party he met two girls. The two standing on their own said hello, he smiled. They had hair as short as Amaka's, wore shiny lipstick and pants so tight they would walk differently if they were wearing something more comfortable.

He watched them examine themselves in the mirror in the arrivals hall, poring over an American magazine with a brown skinned, honey-haired woman on the cover, and talk about a maths teacher who didn't know the answers to her own test. A girl who wore a miniskirt to the evening gig even though she had fat yams on her legs, and a boy who was fine, 'fine *sha*, not attractive,' one of them emphasised. He was turned off by their puerile manners. He bounced.

He looked across the hall and saw someone standing alone waiting for another friend to join her. She wore a dangling earring on one ear and a shiny, false gold stud on the other. She was wearing a mauve silk dress with flashing boho hem, lime-green lattice wedge scandals, a black corduroy with a fly-away collar, and her artificial afro was arranged in a sequence of diagonal cornrows at the front with the rest left freely hanging though tamed with a palmful S-Curl gel.

Framed within this her expression was childlike, a high forehead and slyly vulnerable eyes. Together they displayed an ordinary transient beauty. She was the one that turned heads. He inched himself closer to chat the girl up. Standing up close and in proximity her face revealed shadows, dulled, imperfect first lines.

She was on the far side of youth at a moment in her life when the gradual descent into old age was beginning to show. Chichi had hoped to find a girl to mount that night, he was disappointed this was not his lucky night. However, he wants to replicate this experience and achieve the fantasies he missed the last time. If the party is to happen, they need a mediator to break the impasse.

Like me, the brothers are tired of engaging in recycled conversations time and again, tired of sitting around the apartment chasing their heels. They want their lives back. Now. I have skin hunger for human touch.

This apartment symbolises a break with everything I know. On the one hand, the days blurred into endless identical cycles of sameness. On the other, a sporadic theatre of comedies. There is a rotating cast calling themselves relatives with their small children most of whom are unknown to the brothers, including the loud-talking aunty Tsitsi who frequents this apartment with monotonous regularity. There is the matter of noise, the desperate braying of everyone talking over everyone else, the bad music, the children and dogs, the radios from the frats down to the car stereos in the streets, the shouting mass of hundreds of mouths disagreeing. Its madness.

Everybody's appetite is delicate this morning, except Azu's: he ate his way through three eggs. Chichi sipped coffee and radiated waves of disapproval. I watched in frank admiration.

The apartment sometimes sparkles but most times not so much—Azu is responsible for scrubbing the floors, Chichi does the sweeping, plump up the cushions on the chairs. Everybody takes turns washing plates on days when we remembered to cook. I was included in the plate-washing routine. One morning after we ate, I washed the garri-encrusted plates, Azu picked them off the tray where I had placed them to dry and washed again. We thought his antics were hilarious, we laughed a little bit and then recoiled into our familiar silence.

The silence hanging over the house smothers it, this is a different kind of silence, one that lets me breathe. I have nightmares about the other kind, the silence before the police knock and break down the door to our apartment. In my nightmares, it mixes with shame and grief and so many other things that I cannot name.

The silence is broken only by the whir of the ceiling fan as it sliced through the air once every fifteen minutes or so if we are lucky. The blades of the ceiling fan were encrusted with woolly dust because there had been no power in the apartment for a while or the dust would have flown away as the fan turned.

Although our dining area is spacious, it gives way to an even wider living room. Even so, I felt suffocated. On the off-white walls hanged framed photos of people I did not know bearing down on me. The glass window was moving towards me. Someone needed to break it, and it was not going to be me. That it had been over a month now, I realised with a thrum of anxiety. The flurry of easy-going taunts made me feel a little sad, the kind of private sadness you could conceal from yourself until one day you surfaced and found it waiting.

A directed desire to live gives us a path to drive on, but once we reach the goalpost, a sense of aimlessness befalls us. We realize that the promised land is just a starting point for a long journey, but oftentimes we are unsure of what the next destination is. In other words, we have yet another desire without direction, which means that boredom emerges once again.

Chichi came out from the bathroom and stood at the door fiddling with the back doorknob. Azu understood this gesture was for him. He did not protest but proceeded to the lounge where Ade has been lying for most of the day listening to music on his phone. Azu tried to put on a brave face, but his posture gave him away. He slouched on the couch in the purposeful way a schoolboy slouches in defiance outside the principal's office.

He walked with a permanent forward-canting posture. It is a slouch of someone trying to rebel against whatever authority demands that they sit up and pay attention. It screams annoyance. There was always something vaguely annoying in Azu's expression: subtle snarl, a blank stare, and narrow eyes. I found this both off-putting and a little endearing. Chichi and Azu had never been the sort who traded kind favours, but now they are forced to be in the same enclosure brushing sides constantly they have learned to dig deeper in their reserve to make peace stick.

Azu kicked off his shoes, feeling the cold grit and crunch of dirt under his soles. The wind from the gap under the door squeezed dirt through the hole in his right sock that collected in the big toe he immediately shoved his feet back into the shoes.

I live in a block of apartments with four floors, on each floor there are two doors, each lead to the apartments on that floor. About half of the doors in the apartment building are unknown to me; I am not sure who lives behind them. I have never seen or met the occupants or, talked to them. Some of these doors represent a mystery to me, mystery always excites intrigue and curiosity.

It is a little over four weeks I have been locked inside this tiny flat. I am startled to hear a knock on our door. There she is standing waiting to be let in. I noticed she is pregnant with several months behind her. After she said 'hello,' I looked her in the eye she was chirpy and smiley. She introduced herself to me and we stood at the door engaging in idle chat. Noticing that she intends to go beyond the small chat at the door, I realise I have no choice but to invite her in. She accepts hastily.

Autumn draws fresh cold lines around the neighbourhood. It turns the green leaf into a curling dark apple. There are stories in the streets, many of them already erased by the wind. Many lies sleeping in the cemetery. Some stories persist. They cannot go away or be swept up by the wind. These stories come alive each day in the actions of the people of Kempton. They are truths. I have learned a lot on the short visit from our new neighbour. 'Hey, I am Jill, by the way.' She says elatedly.

Jill is a curiosity. She is wearing blue linen shorts that buttoned to her shirt, her hair is dyed white and stuck to her head like duck fluff. She is a year or two my junior, but she towers over me. As she told me the Kempton stories her brown eyes would lighten and darken; her laugh is sudden and happy. She habitually pulled at a cowlick in the centre of her forehead. I tell her to visit us more often and promise to do the same. 'I love chatting to you.' She says cheerfully. We part ways.

Jill leaves in the same apartment on the ground floor below. I know this because I had to bring her house keys. She left them when visiting earlier. The inside is appalling. Cracks in uneven walls let in a menagerie of insects and rodents and filth that permeated the very air made it impossible to disinfect anything. The bugler gates could not keep out the acrid smoke from a garbage heap smouldering in the ditch outside. The stench seeped in through the one open window. I had a fleeting glimpse of my earlier days as a houseman. Only this made that tumbledown clinic look like state-of-the-art.

End Street, the part of town where our apartment is located is in bad shape. In rainy weather the streets turn to red slop; grass grows on the sidewalks, the courthouse sagged in the square. Somehow, a black dog suffers on a summer's day.

Kempton Park is one of Gauteng's problematic areas during the early phase of coronavirus pandemic, with 20 people dying in three months. What, though, if coronavirus is not just the latest in a series of shocks? Cities that can shrug off a disaster can still fade if their economic base and with it their tax revenues suffers a structural shift. Many businesses have closed thanks to coronavirus; some may never reopen. And the workers to start new ones might be sorely lacking.

Our world has shrunk, cooped up in our positions with fewer demands. It is appeal of submission. The first weeks of the lockdown was a novelty. We baked, exercised. We Zoomed, Googled. The subsequent weeks became harder with frustration built at not being able to exercise outside, not able to socialise especially at not being able to buy Nando's the favourite snack.

Social connections are as important to our flourishing as the need for food, safety, and shelter. Apart from my brothers, I had not spent face-to-face time with anyone else in more than a month and half let alone receive a hug. This is abnormal for me. And I would sit with my knees pressed together, trying hard to keep my face blank, to keep the pride from showing, because Chichi said modesty was important in these times.

And yet even before coronavirus hit, I heard many say lockdown deprived us of social connections. I cannot pretend that social distancing is unprecedented in truth, our social media have been distancing us from each other for years now. Over the last fifteen years, our communities have been growing more and more individualistic, our social connections have been dissolving.

We volunteer less. We are no longer entertain strangers at our homes. And we have fewer and fewer close friends with whom we share the intimate details of our lives. Over the same time that social isolation has increased. We are increasingly denying our social nature and paying a price for it. We have the lockdown to thank for the reminder. This is the reversal of that only harder.

While we were stripped from our normal lives and living on what is essentially was house arrest, this was an opportunity for creativity. We are the most creative when we are free of distraction. We have time to think, imagine and see. That is, if we resist the urge to think about zombies and the idea that if you forget to wash your hands for 20 seconds or sneeze, you will kill a family. Creativity thrives when we have few obligations and lots of free time.

In week six, I found that I have settled into a familiarity with our pared down lives and an adjustment to a new normal I struggle to come to terms with. I struggle with not being active, struggle to form an emotional bond with my invincible captor. Suffering from decision fatigue syndrome is harder. I thought I was ready to push the Crl+Alt+Del button and start over again. Yet, this situation is not in my hands. Nothing is anymore.

I was discovering so many things about myself – good things I had never acknowledged, and unpleasant things I had never faced before. I had a disconcerting sense that something in my life was about to change drastically, it frightens me to the core at the same time it fills me with untold excitement. When it comes to the interactions with my cousins Chichi, Ade and Azu the stress is driven out because I have kept a low profile allowing them to lead.

Kempton Park is twenty kilometres east of Thembisa, awkwardly inland for a town. Stirs with hope and impending upheaval. Some buildings have started to crumble, wind scatters sand from the far south, and political protesters flood the streets with song. Each echo reveals startling insights about what it means to seek connection with those we love, with the place we inhabit and with our own fugitive selves.

Kempton's proportion of professional people ran high at one time: one went there to have one's teeth pulled, one's car fixed, heart listened to, money deposited, soul saved and one's pets vaccinated. On the up-market end of the town stands Glen Marais. There houses have big bathrooms and stairwells. On Sunday night, the mother of the house would line up her children with freshly laundered towels so that they could take their daily bath in hot spice-scented bath tabs and emerge smelling hope.

Kempton Park is mass-transit dependent but not unique in this experience. But the point of a dense town is that it needs density to work. In the morning over twice as many more rush in like a tide, filling up taxi ranks, railway stations and the informal market splashed throughout the town. In the evening, this tide drains back, leaving just a thin residue of a small coterie of shift workers.

The ebb and flow are a trickle at the weekends, and almost dry in December. But it has held its rhythm for more than a sixty-four years. People move slowly here. A day is twenty-four hours long but seems longer. There is no hurry, for there was nowhere to go, nothing to buy and no money to buy it with, nothing to see outside the boundaries of the town square. They amble across the square, shuffle in and out of the surrounding stores, take their time about everything. Doing nothing.

South Africans who live in big metropolitan areas are, on average, 50% more productive than those who live in smaller metros. This holds true even for workers with the same education, experience, working in the same industry. In poor provinces like North West and Northern Cape, the advantages of city life are even greater.

Closing such powerhouses in the face of coronavirus pandemic was a dramatic and expensive miscalculation on the part of government. But it was at least conceptually simple. Reopening them is harder, in large part because of the conflicting requirements of amenity and transport. For almost all cities in Gauteng reopening have seen increased congestion as people who previously used mass transit commute by car and on their own.

If, faced with half-empty offices, service workers do not come back for want of custom, that will add to the commuters' disinclination to return. If the businesses providing services actually go bust waiting for the tide to turn, things will go even worse.

Even if reopening goes well, the hole in the city's finances will be vast. The declines in sales, income and taxes that came with the shutdown will result in a tax-revenue hit over the next few fiscal years.

Compliance with social-distancing measures seem likely to require more space per worker for many months. That will give companies a reason to encourage some workers to stay away some or all the time while not changing the demand for office space much. If workers can conduct their jobs from home permanently, some will leave the city for good.

What is more, an entirely decentralised workforce, however slacked, teamed, hung out and zoomed it might be, cannot capture all the benefits the city has to offer, either for its members in terms of finding better jobs or its employers? Office attendance will become a memory for some, a daily delight for others, and a movable feast for most.

Kempton would have been further away from Thembisa had it not been for the nimble-wittedness of one Sinkie, who in the dawn of history operated an inn where two pig-trails met, the only tavern in the town. Instead, Thembisa and Kempton grew closer, sprawling out from its hub, Sinkie's Tavern. Sinkie is known to reduce his guests to myopic drunkenness, inducing them to bring more cash to his joint.

In the recent years, the inner-city dwellers have grown exponentially. They constitute the majority residents, most of whom are outsiders coming in the main from Nigeria. This town begun its slow decline into drugs, poverty, and ghettoization years shortly after the 2010 FIFA World Cup staged here. Illicit drug peddling is now an established business run by powerful drug cartels and Nigerian underworld syndicates.

Asylum seeking communities found in the inner cities of South Africa are often roundly condemned as *Amakwerekwere ase Nigeria* and *Amakula ase Pakistan*. These communities are hardest hit by the lockdown recently announced by the president. First, we are excluded by government from benefiting from the special coronavirus relief grants offered to all the citizens. Second, we are marginalised by the community we live with and ostracised by our neighbours.

As it is, we have nothing to fall back on. The instincts for survival behove us to fend for ourselves by any means necessary relying on our entrepreneurial skills. We sell everything from food to clothes to cigarettes and drugs. We approached the courts for interim relief, the government said no we do not belong here and ignored court orders. We asked our neighbours for food; they did not have enough to feed themselves let alone to share with refugees they care for nothing. We were on our own.

Something lovely is being lost. It may well be that when the lockdown is over South Africa will no longer be the place it was before coronavirus but one that fills all of us with anxiety. I have a sense of emptiness.

South Africa's old idea of itself unleashed a torrent of negative energy, but the identity that grows up in the shadow of this plague can have the humanity of shared vulnerability, the humility that comes with an understanding of the precariousness of life and a fierce solidarity that emerges during a struggle for humanity. I am not sure if any of them appreciate the loss emerging from the margins.

Maybe I could help attract attention to my writing or publish my story on the website they own. But what do I know about seeing friends massacred, fleeing wars, hiding for their lives in shipping containers and on ill-equipped boats in order to arrive penniless at a windswept shack in the hinterlands of Durban or Cape Town?

The 'exceptional' guy who is asked to sit at the table and explain why riots, why deaths, why the hate, or why a child arrives without a mother or a father, have built-in expiration date. This exceptional person function as a translator of events and rarely as translator of the story, or the translator of loneliness in each place and time in which that story happens.

At meetings and in parties one spends a great deal of time with collaborators – functionaries in service to white privilege – who will step up on your neck to get to the next Afrikan who can explain just what is happening and why. When white South Africa asks an Afrikan man who describes himself as a non-racialist to speak about race, it's almost always from the vantage point of it being a sort of plight and, if those collaborators can listen, what they hear is 'who is an Afrikan in relation to us white people?'

Unlike the people I met in the jungle, I was not so much living in limbo as living with liminality. I was let inside the tent because I had a green bar-coded identity document on me. Maybe it is because I spoke polished English with a refined London accent an envy of many locals.

It is certain my skin complexion had disguised many facts about me, such as that I, my grandfather was born here, and my grandmother was a teacher at Amanzimtoti College a missionary school south of Durban. I was born here but grew up here in UK. Does South Africa accommodate only the light-skinned, handsome, economically successful men and women? I suspect so.

I was also travelling during the time when a multicultural backlash suggesting that the likes of me represented some sort of failed temporary experiment. It feels like the time to reassert my identity has arrived. My new mission. I have no choice but to let a subjective light slip between the cracks and remind everyone who cares to listen that I am not trying to insert myself in their world I am an inextricable part of their world. My experiences are inseparable from theirs.

After Mandela, none of them cared to explain the dilemma they were to face in years to come. Those in the party do not have to deal directly with these new arrivals, did not have to work with them or foster the kind of goodwill it takes to connect with people from neighbouring states; the construct of this human bridge was left to the comrades in government or, as is happening, refuse to construct them.

These new communities of 'refugees' were visible scapegoats to be used at will for all societal failings. South Africa's power, influence and prosperity was reduced progressively instead of looking at complex socio-economic factors behind this, it was easier to blame rising unemployment and a shaken national identity on 'those people in the inner city who looked different to us and spoke weird languages.'

As I look at the rubble of my life, I am reminded of him who said, 'our anxiety does not empty tomorrow of its sorrows, but only empties today of its strength.' This prophet, Charles Spurgeon had hit the nail on the head. But the prose cannot save me now I must stand up and fight like a man. If the old creed grew up in an atmosphere of assumed security, the new one is growing up in an atmosphere of vulnerability and precariousness.

But the more I think about this situation, I recognise that something more profound is going on here. This country is undergoing a permanent shift in national consciousness, a reconstruction of meanings, symbols, and narratives – coronavirus, xenophobia and cancelled 'Black Lives Matter' campaign.

It seems to me this country has lost a sense of safety, the calm confidence that the future is ours, that our institutions are sound or even minimally competent. And if there was any shred of safety left, surely the pandemic has taken it away. We have had threats before, but we have never had smack in the middle of a crisis of confidence, a crisis of authority plus social crisis all at once.

Sekano, the commander of the north sector policing, has ramped up the police presence in Kempton Park area. One way to control unruly, ungovernable 'refugees,' of course, is to remind them that they are guests of a mighty police state. Every club that cracks open a black skull anywhere is proof of that.

Once I learned that Sekano was an Afrikan, we bent in sorrow, or worse, rose with arms high in grief and anger. What has Mandela's country wrought? Were black men in South Africa willing functionaries of a white system? Did black lives not matter to them, then and ever? Kempton Park was not our home, they reminded us; I get that. Was it ever ours?

We are refugees living on borrowed time. Theirs. We would live and die in this amount of space and no more. I have been watching the drama in the darkened living room. And the characters, like well-rehearsed actors in a stale play, have been hitting their marks all too well. The cast varies from staging to staging but generally consisting of local police straining not to swing batons, fire tear gas, or set off stun grenades. To put down the refugee riots police brutality dealt us cruelty unforgivable.

Ragtag crowds of mostly teenagers and 20-somethings flighting tired and recycled slogans and chants from movements long forgotten, their ranks with masked millennials and Gen Xers unable to really articulate clear outcomes for the mass action; scurrying reporters seeking a semblance of combat-action bona fides accompanied by a rotating cast of 'experts' explaining the riveted, unnerved whites and international viewers why what is happening in Kempton is happening at all. I was the object of their scorn.

We generally view rage as an uncontrollable impulse that needs to come out in unmediated forms. But people craft rage, they cultivate rage, and not just as individuals, communities too and find targets to unleash to. I am resistant to the idea that moral philosophy is just self-help dressed in tweed, but as this year lurched from one rage to the next and found myself becoming hoarse from what felt like shouting into a void.

My collection of this year's experiences is something of a workbook. A tool for parsing the more unwieldy parts of the world. If you know how to listen; mourning is our language. The world around us is not the one we had worked hard for but the quiet degraded one that our not-country said we deserved. We cannot keep anything, the elders said, not even ourselves.

Hope dies in this instance. And yet we need to believe that it will come back and attach itself to a new cause – a new love, a new house, something that gives us a sense of purpose, which is ultimately what hope is. Would any of it dismantle the xenophobic tensions I must navigate, that which defines our de-facto underclass, that keep us scavenging for food and clothes, even if it was just a pair of sneakers snatched through the pane of a broken glass?

I do not remember when my family and I moved to Hillbrow, but demonstrations and riots against us were staged. Then, after a time, we moved to Bes Valley riots followed us there too. No place was safe, because wherever we congregated was unsafe. The property laws, economics and widespread xenophobia made us unsafe. We were persona non-grata.

To social workers, who visited us whenever they thought our women were entertaining men and getting paid for it. To shopkeepers, who did not understand that the deprivations of poverty were a rather good incentive for us to take what we had never able to buy. To schoolteachers, who were not paid to care. To a society that demanded our gratitude for the dried gruel at the bottom of the bowl which it tossed us after years of unpaid labour. To the Afrikan brothers whom we wanted to befriend but could not for fear our vulnerability would compound theirs.

As a little boy growing up in Hillbrow, I was tormented by the question of protection, because I too, wanted to be protected. Like any number of Afrikan boys in that neighbourhood, I grew up in a matrilineal society, where I had been taught the power of silence. But how could you not cry out when you could not save yourself because you could not defend yourself?

Although I had something in common with Chichi, Azu and Ade, something else distinguished me from them when black bodies were threatened. The guys who took the chance to protect themselves were the same guys who called me a faggot not so long ago. The silence I was taught as a means of survival cannot be a good thing going forward.

But I know what I would not give up entirely – it is hard to give up. My sense of community. It is not necessarily through acts of physical violence, whether experienced first-hand or by word of mouth that a child is initiated into the contradictions of discriminating society like what I am going through right now.

Rather, it is through brief impersonal encounters, stares, vocal inflections, hostile laughter, or public reversals of private expectations that occur at the stage when children are most perceptive to the world and its wonders. In my world, there is nothing impersonal when it comes to xenophobia, or the will to subjugate the other. Every act of xenophobia is a deeply personal act with the result; the unmooring diminishment of the person who is its target. If you have suffered the kind of erasure like me, you are less likely to know who you are where you live.

I keep seeing the loneliness inherent in the Afrikan child, my refugee status dressed up in self-protective decorum, because if the child can get to my loneliness and articulate it he can also begin to talk about community and why it is needed in life too. My community is my memory.

If I cannot tell my story, who will? Tell me where to begin telling my story, which will have to include my fears and their hate. Shall I begin by showing the collaborators the wounds I have suffered on the auction block of post-apartheid democracy and its culture of denialism? Or should I shut up and learn forgiveness after forgiveness? But can I forgive myself for forgiving? Surely there is another language, a different weight on the soul?

And what will the world look like after this time becomes just another moment in history? Will there be a backlash from the land where those seen as 'refugees' come from? Will South Africa become tired of my refugee status and revert to what it always was dreams and amnesia once the Black Lives Matter ceases to be politically correct, or will they integrate me into the social fabric of this society with empathy without ridiculing me or erasing my presence?

With my life reduced to its foundation, I have had to think hard what it was built on. I ask is this all there is to my story and why my world was burning? Then I remembered this is not my world and this is not my story. It is not even theirs. None of it. In this very instance I started noticing things about life as I saw them from an outsider perspective.

It is the duty of the writer to have a longer memory than the nations. And not only a longer memory but a more precise rendering of events as they happen. The state will only ever record its triumphs, but it will never indict itself for the reasons those things were necessary.

It is the duty of the writer not only to resist such narratives but to ardently counter them, to remind people that a basic truth remains: The conditions that produced our protests have gone unchanged. We must repeat this as though it is the only song we know.

I cannot give in to the alluring narrative of progress, which simply means that today's suffering is slightly less deadly than yesterdays. But where economic deprivation persists, social care is denied, safe housing is in short supply, police kill with impunity, and we are not even provided masks to prevent the spread of deadly coronavirus disease during a global pandemic.

We are, in fact, expected to be the sacrificial lambs on the altar of capitalist profiteering. Black capitalists. What passes for progress is so inadequate as to be itself useless. As writers, we must not say that the fire is coming, but that it was never extinguished in the first place. Life is not a happy thing right now. It is stressful, strange, and upside-down. I am weary with exhaustion by isolation, tired of all the nothing, are you?

Amid crisis and disruption, I crave freedom. Can freedom become a burden too heavy to bear, I ask the president? Is this something I can escape from? Is there not also, besides an innate desire for freedom, an instinctive wish on my part for submission to their rules? If not, how do I account for the attraction which submission has over me? It was Ron Derby who said the following words.

'One thing that has held true through any turbulent time in world history is that periods of crisis come with fracturing societies, heightened divisions where our worst human traits come to the fore. These periods of grave danger come with political choices muddied by our own prejudices against different race groups and foreigners in the battle for survival.'

As much as this is true, we need to remember that these periods come with opportunity. Steering a country away from poor political choices in the main becomes the job of its leading political actors. Perhaps, it is just a question of luck, of whether a country is cursed with the fervour and closed-mindedness of nationalism, bred by fear. Being opportunistic and in truth, brave enough to see a chance for realising reforms that have conflicted with protecting wealth built in what essentially is a corrupted economy.

※ ※

Azu was only 15 when I first heard him sing:
> Babalawo mow a bebe
> Alugbinrin
> Ogun to se fun mi lere kan
> Alugbinrin
> Oni nma ma fowo kenu
> Alugbinrin
> Oni nma ma fese kenu

I do not know the meaning of this song or where he got it from, but he was fond of singing sometime humming in contemplative moods. One time I was in the loo when I heard. 'Kai. You are killing my vibe. Kuro n be. Move, jo! haba!' The last time he sung this song was when we were at a New Year's Eve party and overstayed it.

It has been two years since the cousins hosted a New Year's Party together. Come dusk, the house would be packed; first we ate, then we sat around, listening carefully to one another's tracks, and explaining why that music was important to us. The songs, the music all seemed to come together to fill the vacuum in our lives. Eventually we would drift to bed a few made it through to midnight. The music we chose was always eclectic covering a broad mix of genres – from contemporary to the classics.

Whenever I hear one of those songs, I still remember the person who chose it, and what he told us about it because that's how music works. Unlike literature, musical notes do not mean something concrete the way a word like 'car' or 'house' does. Music goes beyond boundaries of time and consciousness, just as it moves beyond the boundaries of language. It speaks somewhere beneath the skin in an unspeakable language.

Which brings me to my choice of healing songs. We need healing in the situation. The first is a sonata by Bach. As you listen, you find there is room to breathe, it gives a feeling of what others call divinity, a state of serenity and tranquillity. You sense that

Bach has been lonely in his time and very frightened and has used his music to make peace with those feelings. It is full of poise and therefore hope.

Whether it is a soprano voice reaching a high note that my throat fills with ash, or Roberta Flack's soulful six octave voice, I listen. I am right to hurt so much because they too hurt. Music reminds us broken as we sometimes feel, or lost or angry, or full of fear - of a place that is nothing to do with words, and nothing to do with differences. A bigger place that holds us in its embrace.

When I think of Duke Ellington turning off the lights on his band, one by one. It is the happiest ever goodbye, but it also captures something bigger. It tells us we are not up to very much when we standalone, but when we look out for one another and use our skills to help one another, we really are quiet about something. A utopian whole. We played this music at my graduation party and every time I listen to it; I feel incredibly happy and incredibly alone, and I know it is okay to feel such ambiguity. There is room for music to feel many things.

Sunday, 24th May
Virus genesis remains a mystery

According to the testimony of Robert Redfield, the Director of CDC to the USA Foreign Policy Select Committee, the COVID-19 was detected in Wuhan, Hubei province of China, but that does not mean that the novel coronavirus had originated there. It may have originated from elsewhere. To determine the origin of this unknown virus requires, meticulous scientific research instead of wild speculation by ill-advised self-serving politicians. The source of the virus is a scientific issue under investigation. Trust me, we are keen to find out for the sake of future warning system.

There may have been cases of COVID-19 in Los Angeles as early as last December 2019, months before the first known U.S. cases were identified, a new study claim. The study was published in September in the *Journal of Medical Internet Research*.

Without evidence supported by data, no one can claim to know where coronavirus had originated. Connecting a virus with a region serves to fuel xenophobic behaviour. The pandemic influenza of 2009 originated in North America, but it was never called American flu. That is why the WHO named this pandemic COVID-19, which avoids stigmatisation of a region and it has nothing to do with a geographic location, animals, or individuals.

A research team at the Scripps Research Institute has proved their genetic analysis of the novel Coronavirus origins and comparison to available genome sequence data for other known strains of coronavirus proved that this new strain originated through natural processes and has a 96.2% similarity to a bat SARS-related coronavirus.

Scientists in China have successfully sequenced the entire genome of at least 115 samples of the virus. The data strongly suggests that it was initially hosted by an animal before transmitting itself to humans. Bats are the most strongly suspected origin hosts because there is minimal difference between the RNA samples of a bat virus taken in Wuhan and the samples from those hospitalized early in the outbreak.

One of the questions that remains to be answered is where SARS-CoV-2, the virus that causes COVID-19, came from. It is thought the answer involves bats because they harbour a variety of SARS-like viruses. Yunnan, one of China's southernmost provinces, has drawn the attention of virus hunters, as the closest-known relatives of SARS-CoV-2 are found there. But some think the origins of the virus are not to be found in China at all, but rather across the border in Myanmar, Laos, or Vietnam.

This is the hunch of Peter Daszak, head of Eco Health Alliance, an organisation which researches animals that harbour diseases that move into people. Since the outbreak, in 2003, of the original SARS-CoV, scientists have paid close attention to coronaviruses. Dr Daszak says that around 16,000 bats have been sampled and around 100 new SARS-like viruses discovered. Some bats found in China are now known to harbour coronaviruses that seem pre-adapted to infect people.

The chiropteran hosts of these viruses have versions of a protein called ACE2 that closely resemble the equivalent in people. This molecule is used by SARS-like viruses as a point of entry into a cell. That such virologic diversity has so far been found only in China is because few people have looked at bats in countries on the other side of the border. Yet these places are likely to be an evolutionary hotspot for coronaviruses one that mirrors bat diversity.

The horseshoe bats in Yunnan which harbour close relatives of SARS-CoV-2 are found across the region. Other countries are thus likely to have bats with similar viral building blocks. Dr Daszak believes it is quite likely that bats in Myanmar, Laos and Vietnam carry similar SARS-related coronaviruses, maybe a huge diversity of them, and that some of them could be close to SARS-CoV-2.

None of this, though, explains how a virus whose ancestor may be found in South-East Asian bats went on to start a pandemic from central China. China's government has agreed that a mission led by the WHO can visit that country later in 2020 to help answer this question. There is particular interest in how much sampling has been conducted to look for the missing link in places like the wildlife market in Wuhan the first known centre of the outbreak and more generally in farmers, traders and possible intermediate or host species.

Dr Farrar spent 18 years working in Vietnam as the head of an Oxford University research unit. He says people go searching for bats for food and sell them in markets in what is a sophisticated trade that can end up in big cities like Wuhan. Bats can carry a huge diversity of viruses without getting sick and are also more mobile than people realise. As he puts it, bats congregate in huge colonies, and poo everywhere. And then other mammals live off that poo and then act as a mixing vessel for these sorts of viruses.

Support for the idea that something resembling SARS-CoV-2 might have been circulating in the region before the pandemic began also comes from another intriguing observation: the low incidence of COVID-19 in South-East Asia, particularly in Vietnam. John Bell, a professor of Medicine at the University of Oxford, says everyone thought there would be a flood of cases in Vietnam because the country is right across the border from China. Yet Vietnam has reported only 300 in a population of 100m, and no deaths. The country did not have lockdown either, he adds. Nobody could work out what was going on.

One explanation, he suggests, is that Vietnam's population is not as immunologically 'naïve' as has been assumed. The circulation of other SARS-like viruses could have conferred a generalised immunity to such pathogens. So, if a new one emerged in the region, it was able to take hold in the human population only when it travelled all the way to central China where people did not have this natural resistance.

This would tie in with the idea that infection with one coronavirus can provide protection against others, and that even in countries away from the evolutionary cauldron of South-East Asia part of the population may have some protection against the current pandemic. There are suggestions that protection might be conferred mainly via part of the immune system called T-cells which work by killing virus-infected cells rather than via antibodies which work by gumming up pathogens. If that is the case, then serological studies which look at antibodies may be underestimating natural immunity.

As for the mystery of the origin of COVID-19, answers will come when the 34 member scientific team consisting of WHO mission and Chinese experts will start their work in January 2021. One year on, the focus will be on talking to medical staff and clinicians involved in treating patients, parsing medical records, and examining data around the timeline of admissions to determine whether any other cases could retrospectively be identified as COVID-19.

Serological testing on frozen blood samples or plasma could also determine how far back coronavirus antibodies were in the human population. Kamradt-Scott believes it is likely that the virus 'had been circulating previously, or at least it had started circulating in a small community somewhere, but we lacked the diagnostic tools to detect it.'

The day arrived when WHO sent its team to China. Included in that team were 17 Chinese experts, plus seven other experts and support staff from various agencies. They looked at the clinical epidemiology i.e., how Covid-19 spread among people, the molecular epidemiology i.e., the genetic makeup of the virus and its spread, and the role of animals and the environment. As the WHO team began its mission, the question on many people's minds is whether that small community where it all started was in China or elsewhere. Dominic Dwyer, Director of Public Health Pathology, NSW Health Pathology at the Westmead Hospital and University of Sydney wrote a first person account that was published in *The Conversation*. Dominic said.

> As I write, I am in hotel quarantine in Sydney, after returning from Wuhan, China. There, I was the Australian representative on the international World Health Organization's investigation into the origins of the SARS-CoV-2 virus. Much has been said of the politics surrounding the mission to investigate the viral origins of Covid-19. It is easy to forget that behind these investigations are real people. As part of the mission, we met the man who, on December 8, 2019, was the first confirmed Covid-19 case. He has since recovered. We met the husband of a doctor who died of Covid-19 and left behind a young child. We met the doctors who worked in the Wuhan hospitals treating those early Covid-19 cases and learned what happened to them and their colleagues. We witnessed the impact of Covid-19 on many individuals and communities, affected so early in the pandemic, when we did not know much about the virus, how it spreads, how to treat Covid-19, or its impacts. We talked to our Chinese counterparts –

scientists, epidemiologists, doctors – over the four weeks the WHO mission was in China. We were in meetings with them for up to 15 hours a day, so we became colleagues, even friends. This allowed us to build respect and trust in a way you could not necessarily do via Zoom or email. It was in Wuhan, in central China, that the virus, now called SARS-CoV-2, emerged in December 2019, unleashing the greatest infectious disease outbreak since the 1918-'19 influenza pandemic. Our investigations concluded the virus was most likely of animal origin. It probably crossed over to humans from bats, via an as-yet-unknown intermediary animal, at an unknown location. Such "zoonotic" diseases have triggered pandemics before. But we are still working to confirm the exact chain of events that led to the current pandemic. Sampling of bats in Hubei province and wildlife across China has revealed no SARS-CoV-2 to date. We visited the now-closed Wuhan wet market which, in the early days of the pandemic, was blamed as the source of the virus. Some stalls at the market sold "domesticated" wildlife products. These are animals raised for food, such as bamboo rats, civets and ferret badgers. There is also evidence some domesticated wildlife may be susceptible to SARS-CoV-2. However, none of the animal products sampled after the market's closure tested positive for SARS-CoV-2. We also know not all of those first 174 early Covid-19 cases visited the market, including the man who was diagnosed in December 2019 with the earliest onset date. However, when we visited the closed market, it is easy to see how an infection might have spread there. When it was open, there would have been around 10,000 people visiting a day, in close proximity, with poor ventilation and drainage. There is also genetic evidence generated during the mission for a transmission cluster there. Viral sequences from several of the market cases were identical, suggesting a transmission cluster. However, there was some diversity in other viral sequences, implying other unknown or unsampled chains of transmission. A summary of modelling studies of the time to the most recent common ancestor of SARS-CoV-2 sequences estimated the start of the pandemic between mid-November and early December. There are also publications suggesting SARS-CoV-2 circulation in various countries earlier than the first case in Wuhan, although these require confirmation. The market in Wuhan, in the end, was more of an amplifying event rather than necessarily a true ground zero. So we need to look elsewhere for the viral origins. Then there was the "cold chain" hypothesis. This is the idea the virus might have originated from elsewhere via the farming, catching, processing, transporting, refrigeration or freezing of food. Was that food ice cream, fish, wildlife meat? We do not know. It is unproven that this triggered the origin of the virus itself. But to what extent did it contribute to its spread? Again, we do not know. Several "cold chain" products present in the Wuhan market were not tested for the virus. Environmental sampling in the market showed viral surface contamination. This may indicate the introduction of SARS-CoV-2 through infected people, or contaminated animal products and "cold chain" products. Investigation of "cold chain" products and virus survival at low temperatures is still underway. The most politically sensitive option we looked at was the virus escaping from a laboratory. We concluded this was extremely unlikely. We visited the Wuhan Institute of Virology, which is an impressive research facility and looks to be run well, with due regard to staff health. We spoke to the scientists there. We heard that scientists' blood samples, which are routinely taken and stored, were tested for signs they had been infected. No evidence of antibodies to the coronavirus was found. We looked at their biosecurity audits. No evidence. We looked at the closest virus to SARS-CoV-2 they were working on – the virus RaTG13 – which had been detected in caves in southern China where some miners had died seven years previously. But all the scientists had was a genetic sequence for this virus. They had not managed to grow it in culture. While viruses certainly do escape from laboratories, this is rare. So, we concluded it was extremely unlikely this had happened in Wuhan. When I say "we", the mission was a joint exercise between the WHO and the Chinese health commission. In all, there were 17 Chinese and 10 international experts, plus seven other experts and support staff from various agencies. We looked at the clinical epidemiology (how Covid-19 spread among people), the molecular epidemiology (the genetic makeup of the virus and its spread), and the role of animals and the environment. The clinical epidemiology group alone looked at China's records of 76,000 episodes from more than 200 institutions of anything that could have resembled Covid-19 – such as influenza-like illnesses, pneumonia and other respiratory illnesses. They found no clear evidence of the substantial circulation of Covid-19 in Wuhan during the latter part of 2019 before the first case.

Our mission to China was only phase one. We are due to publish our official report in the coming weeks. Investigators will also look further afield for data, to investigate evidence the virus was circulating in Europe, for instance, earlier in 2019. Investigators will continue to test wildlife and other animals in the region for signs of the virus. And we will continue to learn from our experiences to improve how we investigate the next pandemic. Irrespective of the origins of the virus, individual people with the disease are at the beginning of the epidemiology data points, sequences and numbers. The long-term physical and psychological effects – the tragedy and anxiety – will be felt in Wuhan, and elsewhere, for decades to come.

Friday 17th July
In a year this is what we knew

The first documented case of COVID-19 was reported in January. Yet health officials had only a feint idea of how the novel coronavirus spread, who the disease affected most, and how best to combat transmission and provide treatment. Public messaging on the seriousness of the virus was often conflicting, confusing at the best of times, including the early advice not to wear masks. Eight months later, scientists think they have a firm handle on how the virus spreads and what should be done to get the pandemic under control.

Excerpt even this optimism was guessing work at best. COVID-19 has rewritten the book on infectious diseases. Doctors did not know that patients who were previously infected by the virus could be re-infected again by the same strain of virus. This evidence came to light in August. Treating the virus has proven especially difficult because it causes multiple complications affecting nearly every organ system. For COVID-19, using drug combinations in lieu of single-drug therapy was essential. A team at the National University of Singapore using an AI-based platform to help accelerate the discovery of optimal combinations of existing drugs that might be effective against COVID-19.

Here are some things we know about COVID-19 now that we did not know in January. COVID-19 spreads much faster than the original SARS, infecting more than ten times the number of people. The current theory is that the novel Coronavirus has a special spike protein that binds to a cell membrane via an enzymatic activation.

Through genomic analysis scientists have learned that the spike protein has a site activated by human cell enzymes called furin, which is found in a wide variety of human tissues. So, the virus can attack multiple organs simultaneously. The activation site seems to allow easier entry into cells for this strain and could potentially influence the stability and transmission rate of the virus.

At first, it was thought the COVID-19 was caught only through touching of contaminated surfaces but new evidence, according to Kimberly Prather of the University of California, San Diego has shown that coronavirus pathogen travels through the air too, the nano particles. 'A lot of evidence has pointed to aerosol transmission of respiratory virus. Influenza can be passed through the air, as can the virus that causes COVID-19. They float on air currents. It takes them hours to settle.

Aerosol can accumulate, remain infectious indoor for hours and be easily inhaled into the lungs.

The virus can become airborne within tiny, suspended droplets called aerosols and infect people beyond two metres, especially in indoor spaces, where the aerosols are trapped and build up. After months of accumulating evidence, WHO finally agreed with researchers that the risk outdoors is lower, but not zero.

After months of scientific study and discussion including some contradictory if not confusing public communication, the experts agree that COVID-19 is a two-phase disease: in the early phase, virus pathology dominates; and in the later phase, immunopathology drives disease.

What it means is that COVID-19's many ways of spreading vex all but the most stringent efforts to control transmission, particularly indoors. Therefore, health experts implore people to avoid large crowds, observe physical distancing, wear masks inside and outside, and continue vigilant handwashing.

Early advice emphasized handwashing, disinfecting surfaces, and sneezing into your elbow, on the assumption that the coronavirus spread mostly through handshakes, contact with infected surfaces, and through close contact with infectious people within two metres.

In the pandemic's early months, health officials stressed handwashing and social distancing, while discouraging masks, for three reasons: There was an extreme shortage of medical-grade masks for health care professionals; the primary means of spread hadn't been conclusively determined; and outbreaks existed only in pockets, having not yet spread to all provinces or communities.

Now the science of how to slow the pandemic has been settled. It is safe to say that every health expert now recommends face masks. Beyond face coverings, health experts advise people to avoid large indoor gatherings, especially at nonessential venues like bars; provide much more widespread testing with quicker results, paired with contact tracing; mandate physical distancing for public places that remain open.

Hand washing and social distancing are the most basic measures of reducing transmission and slowing the pandemic but only when a significant portion of the population follows this protocol. This means that, until we can contain and mitigate the spread, every individual must do their part to stay home, wash their hands thoroughly, avoid touching their face. As we do so, this virus will be stopped in its tracks. Importantly, we will also gain a better understanding of how to handle the next pandemic when it inevitably occurs.

'We truly have great knowledge [of] how we can control the virus,' says Yonatan Grad, MD, an assistant professor of immunology and infectious diseases at Harvard T.H. Chan School of Public Health. What it means is that science has been largely ignored or applied half-heartedly by government and unless something changes, experts do not expect the pandemic to let up.

COVID-19 affects the whole body, not just the lungs. For several weeks, the Centre for Infectious Diseases held firm to the notion that the three recognizable symptoms of COVID-19 were fever, cough, and shortness of breath. By February, studies showed that the virus caused body aches, nausea, and diarrhoea in some people. Then came news of anosmia, the loss of smell. We learned of COVID toe, possible brain infections causing dizziness and confusion, and a severe reaction by the immune system leading to blood clots, heart attacks, and other organ failures.

We already know that viruses such as measles, mumps and meningitis can cause hearing loss and coronavirus can damage the nerves that carry information to and from the brain. The concept that's emerging is that this is not a respiratory illness alone, this is a respiratory illness to start with, but it is actually a vascular illness that kills people through its involvement of the vasculature.

Eight months into the pandemic, there is now a growing body of evidence to support the theory that the novel coronavirus can infect blood vessels. If you start to put all of the data together that's emerging, it turns out that this virus is probably a vasculotropic virus, meaning that it affects the blood vessels, which could explain not only the high prevalence of blood clots, strokes, and heart attacks, but also provide an answer for the diverse set of head-to-toe symptoms that have emerged says Mandeep Mehra, MD, medical director of the Brigham and Women's Hospital Heart and Vascular Centre.

In a paper published in April in the scientific journal *The Lancet*, Mehra and a team of scientists discovered that the SARS-CoV-2 virus can infect the endothelial cells that line the inside of blood vessels. Endothelial cells protect the cardiovascular system, and they release proteins that influence everything from blood clotting to the immune response. In the paper, the scientists showed damage to endothelial cells in the lungs, heart, kidneys, liver, and intestines in people with Covid-19.

A respiratory virus infecting blood vessel cells and circulating through the body is virtually unheard of. Influenza viruses like H1N1 are not known to do this, and the original SARS virus, a sister coronavirus to the current infection, did not spread past the lung. Other types of viruses, such as Ebola or Dengue, can damage endothelial cells, but they are different from viruses that typically infect the lungs.

Benhur Lee, MD, a professor of microbiology at the Icahn School of Medicine at Mount Sinai, says the difference between SARS and SARS-CoV-2 likely stems from an extra protein each of the viruses requires to activate and spread. Although both viruses dock onto cells through ACE2 receptors, another protein is needed to crack open the virus so its genetic material can get into the infected cell.

The additional protein the original SARS virus requires is only present in lung tissue, but the protein for SARS-CoV-2 to activate is present in all cells, especially endothelial cells. Blood vessel damage could also explain why people with pre-existing conditions like high blood pressure, high cholesterol, diabetes, and heart disease are at a higher risk for severe complications from a virus that is supposed to just infect the lungs. All those diseases cause endothelial cell dysfunction, and the additional damage and inflammation in the blood vessels caused by the infection could push them over the edge and cause serious problems.

What it means is that 'Physicians need to think of COVID-19 as a multisystem disease,' says Aakriti Gupta, MD, a resident at Columbia University Irving Medical Centre. Gupta and her colleagues published a review of COVID-19's effects July 20 in the journal Nature Medicine. 'There's a lot of news about clotting, but it's also important to understand that a substantial proportion of these patients suffer kidney, heart, and brain damage,' she says.

Covid-19 stands out for both the scale of its global impact and the apparent randomness of its many symptoms. Physicians have struggled to understand the disease and come up with a unified theory for how it works. Then on the ninth month of the pandemic, the Summit supercomputer at Oak Ridge National Lab in Tennessee set about crunching data on more than 40,000 genes from 17,000 genetic samples to better understand COVID-19. When Summit was done, researchers analysed the results.

It was, in the words of Dr. Daniel Jacobson, lead researcher and chief scientist for computational systems biology at Oak Ridge, a eureka moment. The computer had revealed a new theory about how COVID-19 impacts the body. This was called the *bradykinin hypothesis*. The hypothesis provides a model that explains many aspects of disease including some of its most bizarre symptoms. It also suggests 10-plus potential treatments. Jacobson's group published their results in a paper in the journal *eLife*.

According to the team's findings, a COVID-19 infection generally begins when the virus enters the body through ACE2 receptors in the nose. The virus then proceeds to enter cells in other places where ACE2 is also present such as the intestines, kidneys, and heart. Once COVID-19 has established itself in the body, things start to get bad. According to this group, the data analysed shows that COVID-19 is not content to simply infect cells that already express ACE2 receptors. Instead, it actively hijacks the body's systems, tricking it into upregulating ACE2 receptors in places where they are usually expressed at low or medium levels, including the lungs.

The renin angiotensin system controls aspects of the circulatory system, including the body's levels of a chemical called bradykinin, which helps to regulate blood pressure. According to the analysis, when the virus tweaks the renin, it causes the body's mechanisms for regulating bradykinin to go in the wrong direction. Bradykinin receptors are re-sensitised, and the body stops breaking down bradykinin and accumulates instead.

The result, the researchers say, is to release a massive build-up of bradykinin in the body. It is this chemical storm that is ultimately responsible for many of COVID-19's deaths. Jacobson's team says in their paper that 'the pathology of COVID-19 is likely the result of Bradykinin storms rather than cytokine storms, which had been previously thought to be responsible for COVID-19 deaths, but that the two may be linked.' There were other papers that previously identified bradykinin storms as a possible cause of the pathologies.

As bradykinin builds up in the body, it dramatically increases vascular permeability making the blood vessels leaky. This aligns with recent clinical data, which increasingly views COVID-19 primarily as a vascular disease, rather than a respiratory one. But the disease still has a massive effect on the lungs. As blood vessels start to leak due to a bradykinin storm, the lungs fill with fluid. Immune cells also leak out into the lungs causing inflammation.

Another insidious trick, through another pathway it increases production of hyaluronic acid (HLA) in the lungs. When this combines with fluid leaking into the lungs, it forms a hydrogel, which can fill the lungs in some patients. It is like trying to breathe through Jelly. Its horrendous.

This may explain why ventilators have proven less effective in treating advanced COVID-19 than doctors originally had hoped. It reaches a point where regardless of how much oxygen you pump in, it does not work because the alveoli in the lungs are filled with this hydrogel. Patients can suffocate even while receiving full breathing support.

The bradykinin hypothesis also extends to many of disease's effects on the heart. About one in five hospitalized patients have damage to their hearts, even if they never had cardiac problems before. Some of this is likely due to the virus infecting the heart directly through its ACE2 receptors. But the renin also controls aspects of cardiac contractions and blood pressure. According to the study, bradykinin storms could create arrhythmias and low blood pressure, which have been seen in some patients.

The bradykinin hypothesis also accounts for COVID-19's neurological effects, which are some of the most surprising and concerning elements of the disease. These symptoms which include dizziness, seizures, delirium, and stroke are present in as many as half of hospitalized patients. According to MRI studies in France revealed that many patients have evidence of leaky blood vessels in their brains.

Bradykinin especially at high levels can lead to a breakdown of the blood-brain barrier this barrier acts as a filter between the brain and the rest of the circulatory system. It lets in nutrients while keeping out toxins and pathogens and keeping the brain's internal environment tightly regulated.

If bradykinin storms cause the blood-brain barrier to break down, this could allow harmful cells and compounds into the brain, leading to inflammation, potential brain damage. It has been reported that bradykinin would indeed be likely to increase the permeability of the blood-brain barrier. In addition, similar neurological symptoms have been observed in other diseases that result from an excess of bradykinin.

Increased bradykinin levels could also account for other common COVID-19 symptoms. ACE inhibitors a class of drugs used to treat high blood pressure have a similar effect on the renin system as COVID-19, increasing bradykinin levels. In fact,

Jacobson and his team note in their paper that 'the virus... acts pharmacologically as an ACE inhibitor' directly mirroring the actions of these drugs.

By acting like an ACE inhibitor, COVID-19 may be causing the same effects that hypertensive patients sometimes get when they take blood pressure drugs. ACE inhibitors are known to cause a dry cough and fatigue, the same symptoms of COVID-19. The similarities between ACE inhibitor side effects and COVID-19 symptoms strengthen the bradykinin hypothesis, the researchers say.

The bradykinin hypothesis explains several other seemingly bizarre symptoms. The team speculate that leaky vasculature caused by bradykinin storms could be responsible for COVID toes, a condition involving swollen, bruised toes that some patients experience. Bradykinin can also mess with the thyroid gland, which could produce the thyroid symptoms recently observed in some patients.

The researchers note that some aspects of the renin angiotensin system are sex-linked, with proteins for several receptors such as one called TMSB4X located on the X chromosome. This means that women would have twice the levels of this protein than men a result borne out by the researchers' data. This could explain the lower incidence of mortality in women.

The bradykinin hypothesis contributes to a better understanding and adds novelty to the existing literature according to scientists who peer-reviewed Jacobson's team paper. It predicts nearly all the disease's symptoms and further suggests new treatments for the disease.

Several drugs target aspects of the renin and are already FDA approved to treat other conditions like *danazol*, *stanozolol*, and *ecallantide*, reduce bradykinin production and could potentially stop a deadly bradykinin storm. Drugs like *icatibant*, reduce bradykinin signalling and could blunt its effects once it is already in the body.

Other compounds could treat symptoms associated with bradykinin storms. *Hymecromone*, for example, could reduce hyaluronic acid levels, potentially stopping deadly hydrogels from forming in the lungs. And *timbetasin* could mimic the mechanism that the researchers believe protects women from more severe infections. All these potential treatments are speculative, of course, and would need to be studied in a controlled environment more broadly.

From the start, COVID-19 was clearly more dangerous for older people, ravaging nursing homes and long-term care facilities, which have accounted for more than 40% of deaths as of early June. An impression developed that younger adults and children were not at risk. Now the risk of death in children and teens is low, 'but it is not nil,' William Hanage, PhD, an associate professor of epidemiology at Harvard T.H. Chan School of Public Health, says. And the risk rises consistently with age. These are the numbers of known COVID-19 deaths in the United States by age group, through July 15:

<1: 9
1–4: 8

5–14: 14
15–24: 157
25–34: 844
35–44: 2,169
45–54: 6,021
55–64: 14,693
65–74: 25,268
75–84: 32,066
85+: 40,125

Salata, the Case Western doctor, sees disturbing trends emerging in younger Covid-19 patients at his university hospital. "The most remarkable thing for me is the fact that we are learning of the catastrophic consequences of this viral infection from strokes in younger persons, multisystem inflammatory syndrome in children, cardiac and renal complications, and the long-lasting consequences of symptoms related to a post-Covid syndrome," Salata tells Elemental.

What it means is that 'no age group gets out of this without risk,' Hanage says. And now with the perspective of time, it is becoming clear that some proportion of infections can leave people in any age group with chronic effects. Further, he and other experts say, when the disease builds in younger populations, as it has been doing in dramatic fashion since late May, it then inevitably infects more older people, leading to the rising number of daily deaths we now see.

The typical COVID-19 patient got younger. The most important COVID-19 story right now may be the age shift. The median age of new COVID-19 cases fell from 65 in March to 35 in August. Young adults getting sick during this time were responsible for driving the surge. If the latest surge is concentrated among younger people, that explained the declining death count. Young people are much less likely to die from this disease, even if they face other health risks.

International data from South Korea, Spain, China, and Italy suggest that the COVID-19 case-fatality rate for people older than 70 is 100 times greater than for those younger than 40. The youth shift seems very real, but what is behind it is harder to say. Maybe older people are being more cautious about avoiding crowded indoor spaces. Maybe news reports of young people packing themselves into bars explain the youth spike, since indoor bars are designed to spread the virus. Or maybe government rushed to reopen the economy pushed young people into work environments that got them sick.

The people in the service economy and the retail industry, they tend to be young, and they cannot work remotely. No matter the cause, interpreting the youth surge as good news would be a mistake. Young people infected with COVID-19 still face extreme dangers — and present real danger to their close contacts and their community.

Young people who feel fine can still contract long-term organ damage, particularly to their lungs. They can pass the disease to more vulnerable people, who end up in the hospital; a youth surge could easily translate into a broader uptick some weeks from now. And the sheer breadth of the youth surge could force businesses to shut down, throwing millions more people into limbo or outright unemployment.

The virus ignores seasons. Because heat and humidity reduce the virulence of influenza and some other viruses, slowing their spread in summer, there had been speculation that the novel coronavirus might similarly subside, but outbreaks in March in the Southern Hemisphere, when it was warm there, largely dashed those hopes.

Now, if heat and humidity have any seasonal dampening effect on this virus, it is clearly minor. Rising case numbers across the U.S. Sunbelt in June and July provide very abundant evidence that heat is not going to help the virus go away.' Hanage says.

What this means therefore is that there will likely be a huge reservoir of infected people heading into fall, so new infections could surge even more rapidly as colder weather forces people into more crowded indoor situations. That surge would coincide with the expected seasonal rise in flu cases, potentially overloading health care systems.

The COVID-19 death rate remains somewhat elusive, largely because the documented number of infections is a gross undercount. The actual case count nationwide is now thought to be about 10 times higher than the official tally, according to a study published July 21 in *JAMA* Internal Medicine. That estimate is in line with previous scientific speculation.

What it means is that per infection, this virus is about five times as dangerous as flu. Hanage says. How high is that? 'It is plenty high enough to kill a very large number of people when you consider that this is a pandemic virus for which there is not really any immunity in the population and we would expect it to end up infecting a large fraction of the population,' he says.

Muddled messaging all along and lack of a national plan led to patchwork policies that in many countries largely ignored science and statistics. The United States leads the world in COVID-19 deaths, with 4.2% of the global total.

The lockdown, which aimed to flatten the curve and buy time to develop a coherent mitigation strategy, tools, and supplies, were wasted, at great cost economic cost. The sheer number of infections has now spiralled beyond the point where voluntary mask-wearing and social distancing alone will get the pandemic under control.

People spread the coronavirus unwittingly. On January 21, 2020, when there were 300 known infections in China and none in South Africa, health officials were already getting a sense of the looming global threat, a sense that quickly turned to panic. 'It's transmissible but only with time would they realize why. An important thing we have learned is the role of pre-symptomatic transmission and transmission from people who are only mildly ill.

Meanwhile, the extent to which small children catch, carry, and spread COVID-19 remains unclear, in part because kids have been largely sequestered, and because they're thought to have milder symptoms in most cases, so their infections may often go unnoticed. Hanage has looked over the studies and offers this estimate. 'Younger children are, roughly speaking, about half as likely to become infected in a contact as adults are, maybe a little bit less likely to transmit, but that's not clear.'

People who are not aware they have the virus but are infectious can cause superspreaders events, which infect dozens of people at once. In recent weeks, the spread has been led by younger adults crowding bars and other places where masks have been anathema. Experts think that about 80% of COVID-19 infections are caused by about 20% of infected individuals.

The phenomenon known as 'long COVID' could be a combination of four different syndromes affecting the body at the same time, according to a study by the UK's National Institute for Health Research (NIHR). Long COVID refers to people suffering from recurring symptoms months after they first contracted the virus. The NIHR study said some 60,000 people could be living with long COVID in the UK.

Researchers say those still suffering from symptoms after seven months of infection could be under the grip of post-viral fatigue syndrome, post-intensive care syndrome, permanent organ damage and long-term COVID syndrome. There is no evidence to suggest that children are exempt from long COVID, or that people who were asymptomatic or avoided serious health problems with the virus will not suffer the long-term complications. The symptoms of long COVID include brain fog, stress, and anxiety.

The study's author Dr. Elaine Maxwell said patients can experience a rollercoaster of symptoms that move around the body. She added: The list of symptoms is huge and covers every part of the body and brain. We believe that the term long COVID is being used as a capsule for more than one syndrome, possibly up to four. People without a clear diagnosis told us they're often not believed by health services."

She said there "are people who never had any support in hospital, never had a test, have no record of ever having had COVID-19, except their own personal history. They may be suffering far more than somebody who was ventilated for several weeks. Maxwell added that the number of people with long-term COVID-19 symptoms is likely to increase amid the return of heavy hospitalizations and a second spike of infections.

Dozens of vaccine candidates are in various stages of testing by different companies and research groups. Optimism was recently boosted when three separate groups in China, at Oxford University, and in the United States announced successful early trials, each generating an immune response to the novel coronavirus and appearing to be safe.

'Absolutely, for sure,' a successful vaccine will be developed for COVID-19, says Barry Bloom, PhD, an immunologist and infectious disease expert at Harvard T.H. Chan School of Public Health and we will get more than one.' With each company able to ramp up production of its own vaccine separately, that would mean more total doses would be available sooner. A vaccine needs to be just 50% effective to make it to market, Bloom says. Expecting a vaccine being administered to the public by March 2021 'is not out of the realm of possibility.'

Causal connections in society and history are hard to trace, I believe this is an inadequate diagnosis. Science has now helped us understand the relationship between animals and viral epidemics in recent history. We know that outbreak such as HIV, MERS, Zika, Bird and Swine flu, Ebola, and Coronavirus we should not have contracted. Humans have upset the harmony and delicate balance between nature, habitat, and the animal kingdom.

The unprecedented consumption seen during the 21st century has affected this relationship in ways that are harmful for the ecosystem. As the Sars, H1N1, Ebola, and Mers epidemics have shown us, it is inevitable that novel viruses will continue to spill over from nature. Because of global warming, we can expect much more virulent epidemics. As soon as the coronavirus has been defeated, strategies will have to be developed to deal with the potential for the next pandemic, which are invisible but infinitely dangerous. Pandemics ends when the pathogens causing them runs out of individuals to infect.

The question of equilibrium balancing use with renewal, with its impact on ecosystems is key to understanding the sudden eruption of epidemics. Nature is groaning against humanity; animals are pushing back against mistreatment at the hands of humans with deadly consequences.

I suspect that with the continued encroachment of humans into habitats of other critters and the destruction of the environment, we will be coming into contact with more of the several kinds of viruses, some of which will spread easily like SARS-nCOV-2, some not so much as with viruses like Nipah (from pig) and Hendra (from horse). Life on earth depends on balanced interactions between people, the natural environment, animals, and their economic systems.

Then we scientists discovered something big. Our genetic makeup makes us to fall sick easy or not get sick at all. As a geneticist has spent much time studying people with unusual traits of resilience to illnesses. His initial instinct was to wonder whether there were people who the virus was unable to infect. Bobe's idea was to try and find entire families where multiple generations had suffered severe cases of Covid-19, but one individual was asymptomatic to understand the genetic factors at play and identify genetic factors behind resilience.

Researchers have identified an association between type O and rhesus negative blood groups, and a lower risk of severe disease. But while scientists have hypothesised that people with certain blood types may naturally have antibodies capable of recognising some aspect of the virus, the precise nature of the link remains unclear.

Scientists have probed the human genome for clues as to why some people become unexpectedly and severely ill when infected by common viruses ranging from herpes to influenza. In every infectious disease, you can always find outliers who become severely ill, because they have genetic mutations which make them susceptible.

Mayana Zatz, director of the Human Genome Research Centre at the University of São Paulo has identified 100 couples, where one person got Covid-19 but their partner was not infected. Her team is now studying them in the hope of identifying genetic markers of resilience. "The idea is to try and find why some people who are heavily exposed to the virus do not develop Covid-19 and remain serum negative with no antibodies.

Zatz is also analysing the genomes of 12 centenarians who have only been mildly affected by the coronavirus, including one 114-year-old woman in Recife who she believes to be the oldest person in the world to have recovered from Covid-19. While Covid-19 has been particularly deadly to the older generations, elderly people who are remarkably resistant could offer clues for new ways to help the vulnerable survive future pandemics.

In the 1960s, already scientists had discovered our cells have an inbuilt alarm system to alert the rest of the body when it's being attacked by a new virus. When a virus enters a cell, the infected cell makes proteins called type one interferons, which it releases outside the cell. All the surrounding cells receive that signal, and they prepare to fight that virus. Then cells will make enough type one interferon that it's released into the bloodstream, and so the entire body knows that it's under attack.

Sometimes genetic flaws mean that this system malfunctions. In 2015, scientists identified mutations in young healthy people which led to them developing severe pneumonia from influenza because there was no interferon response. If the alarm is silenced, then the virus can spread and proliferate much faster within the body.

It appears this also plays a role in making some people unexpectedly vulnerable to COVID-19. Series of papers compared 987 outliers in COVID-19 patients who developed severe pneumonia who were either younger than 50, or older than 50 and without any co-morbidities to asymptomatic patients. Around 3.5% had a major gene mutation which made it impossible for them to generate an interferon response. Another 10% were found to have self-targeted antibodies in their blood, known as autoantibodies, which bind to interferon proteins and remove them from the bloodstream before the alert signal goes out to the rest of the body.

Autoantibodies play a key role in serious cases of COVID-19 by shutting down the body's ability to defend itself against viruses. There's evidence a significant number of patients with severe disease are making unusual amounts and types of autoantibodies. But autoantibodies and mutations that block interferon account for 14% of patients. For the remaining 86%, geneticists believe their vulnerability arises from a network of genetic interactions when a virus strikes. Only a small number get severely infected because they have a mutation in one main gene. Most patients are following a more complex model in which many genes are co-operating between them, leading to susceptibility to severe COVID-19.

Scientists at the University of Edinburgh have studied the genomes of 2,700 patients in intensive care units across the UK and compared them with those of healthy volunteers. They found that people vulnerable to COVID-19 have five genes linked to interferon response and susceptibility to lung inflammation active than the general population. This combination means that the virus is able to spread more easily through their body, and they are more likely to incur lung damage as a result. This may explain why those with type A blood groups seem to have a higher risk factor for severe disease. Says Erola Pairo-Castineira, one of the geneticists who led the study.

Studying the COVID-19 outliers is providing insights into other mysteries of the pandemic, such as why men are more susceptible than women. After puberty, men have an increase in testosterone, which downregulates all the interferon genes. So, for men who already have a defect in these genes, this is going to make them far more vulnerable to a virus.

Wednesday, 16th August
Afrika least harmed. Kanjani?

The United Nations Economic Commission for Africa predicted that in April up to 300,000 deaths if the virus could not be contained on the continent. The Africa Centres for Disease Control and Prevention was reporting in December 2020 63,300 deaths for a population of 1.2 billion. Of all the Afrikan countries, South Africa was the most affected with 30,000 deaths by end of December on the count of the second wave. Her immediate neighbours: Eswatini, Lesotho, Botswana, Mozambique, Namibia, and Zimbabwe combined had by August registered 456 deaths. There are at least two countries that had no coronavirus infections and at least four countries that did not register a single death.

The national mortality rate excluding excess deaths had remained below 2% with a recovery rate of 90%. The SA Medical Research Council reported excess death to be around 39000 in 2020. Even so, for a population of 61 million this is a low mortality rate whether one is looking at the official figures alone or in combination with excess death.

The Gauteng province is the second biggest region in terms of population size. It is home to approximately 12,3 million citizens. By 1st July, the province had registered only 256 confirmed COVID-19 deaths. The same number of deaths recorded for flu related illness in previous years. When the province peaked in the first wave by end of December the number of deaths had been around the 5422 mark, the most in the country. In the end, the national experience was that nine out of ten coronavirus infected patients recovered fully. Overall, Africa defied the doomsday predictions. Why that might be the case is unclear and what explains this low mortality remains a mystery?

However, the African CDC says there has been no indication that many COVID-19 deaths have been missed. Yet antibody surveys suggest far more Afrikans have been infected with the coronavirus – a discrepancy that puzzled scientist around the world. 'We do not have an answer,' said Sophie Uyoga at the Kenya Medical Research Institute.

After testing more than 3000 blood donors, Uyoga and colleagues estimated in a preprint that one in 20 Kenyans aged 15 to 64—or 1.6 million people—has antibodies to SARS-CoV-2, an indication of past infection. That would put Kenya on a par with Spain in mid-May when that country had 27,000 official COVID-19 deaths. Kenya's official toll stood at 100 when the study ended. And Kenya's hospitals are not reporting high numbers of people with COVID-19 symptoms.

Other antibody studies have yielded similarly surprising findings. From a survey of 500 asymptomatic health care workers in Blantyre, Malawi, immunologist Kondwani Jambo of the Malawi–Liverpool Wellcome Trust Clinical Research Programme and colleagues concluded that up to 12.3% of them had been exposed to the coronavirus. Based on those findings and mortality ratios for COVID-19 elsewhere, they estimated that reported number of deaths in Blantyre at the time, 17, was eight times lower than expected.

Scientists who surveyed about 10,000 people in two cities in Mozambique, Nampula and Pemba, found antibodies to SARS-CoV-2 in 3% to 10% of participants, depending on their occupation; market vendors had the highest rates, followed by health workers. Yet in Nampula, a city of approximately 750,000, a mere 300 infections had been confirmed at the time. Mozambique only has 16 confirmed COVID-19 deaths. Yap Boum of Epicentre Africa, the research and training arm of Doctors Without Borders, says many people in Cameroon have COVID-19 antibodies as well.

What explains the gap between antibody data and the official toll? Part of the reason may be that Africa misses many more cases than other parts of the world because it tests far less. Overall, testing for COVID-19 cases has been comparatively limited on the continent, which could be contributing to lower case numbers. South Africa, which has the highest testing rate in the region, was only performing 0.68 tests a day per 1,000 people in mid-December. Kenya tests about one in every 10,000 inhabitants daily. Nigeria tests one out of every 50,000 people per day. Even many people who die from COVID-19 may not get a proper diagnosis. Even so, you should still expect an overall rise in mortality which was not the case.

There would be multiple explanations for lower numbers, not one solid reason, says Cape Town-based independent clinical epidemiologist Dr Nandi Siegfried. It could be due to a lower average age, a more favourable climate, or fewer co-morbidities on the continent each offers an imperfect defence, which taken cumulatively, contributes to an overall protective effect.

Africa's youthfulness may protect it. In Kenya and Malawi, it is 20 and 18, respectively. Young people around the world are far less likely to get severely ill or die from the virus. And the population in Kenya's cities, where the pandemic first took hold, skews even younger than the country, says Thumbi Mwangi, an epidemiologist at the University of Nairobi.

Many African countries have no infrastructure, but they also have longstanding experience with infectious disease, more exposure to other coronaviruses that cause little more than colds in humans, which may provide some defence against COVID-19. Some epidemiologists suspect that the close contact with other people and regular exposure to different pathogens like malaria or other infectious diseases could make

Afrikans more resistant to the worst forms of COVID-19. Boum Barasa, on the other hand, suspects genetic factors protect the Afrikan population from severe disease.

South African epidemiologist Siegfried could point to one factor in the continent's low COVID-19 mortality rate, it would be that Africa's median age is 19 years old. 'We don't have many people over the age of 50. It seems logical that a relatively youthful population would result in a lower toll. The fact that diabetes, obesity and hypertension, the comorbidities that make COVID-19 more deadly, are also less common among the continent's population than they are in other parts of the world. South Africa is an exception to this generalisation. Siegfried missed one crucial factor however in the defence against the coronavirus infections, Vitamin D. The immune system and our vitamin D blood level have a close relationship.

Recent studies have shown that vitamin D is the single most important immune shield against coronavirus. Vitamin D is making the immune system strong by triggering the release of cathelicidin and defensins, two groups of antiviral polypeptides that kill viruses like the COVID-19 coronavirus. Patients that have encountered Covid-19 coronavirus are more likely to survive if blood level is up to the higher range of normal, between 50 and 80 ng/mL. Because of all these qualities vitamin D lowers the risk of significantly. It not only minimizes the risk of hospitalization but also lowers mortality from.

The American research group outlined 3 mechanisms of how vitamin D works.
1. Maintaining tight epithelial junctions making it more difficult for the Covid-19 coronavirus to penetrate.
2. "Killing enveloped viruses through induction of cathelicidin and defensins." These powerful antiviral polypeptides can kill viruses that have invaded the bloodstream within 1 to 2 days.
3. And reducing production of proinflammatory cytokines by the innate immune system, thereby reducing the risk of a cytokine storm leading to pneumonia.

The COVID-19 virus appears to dissipate quickly outside, where infectious respiratory droplets and aerosols can be easily dispersed, which is why socialising, when necessary, is done outside. With a few exceptions. Africa's winters are moderate to mild this means that much of life tends to be as is the case lived outside. Public transport excerpt in urban cities is generally poor in the continent this means that Africans do not travel much between countries and cities, minimizing the risk of exposure.

If tens of millions of Africans have already been infected, that raises the question of whether the continent should try for herd immunity without a vaccine, Boum says the idea of letting the virus run its course to allow the population to become immune, perhaps while shielding the most vulnerable is controversial. That might be preferable over control measures that cripple economies and could harm public health more in the long run. 'Maybe Africa can afford it,' given the apparent low death rate, he says.

According to research findings on the COVID-19 genome, the virus mutates 24 times each year or twice per month, which is like the mutation rate of the flu. However, novel Coronavirus has a longer genome than the flu, meaning there are fewer mutations per base. This is normal and to be expected, as viral mutations are a natural part of the lifecycle of a virus. But what does this mean? Well, science says these mutations mean that we are all experiencing a slightly different coronavirus from country to country.

We now know from all the compiled research that there have been several different versions of the novel coronavirus throughout the course of this pandemic. But how does this happen? Think of the small genetic code changes in the virus as fingerprints used by geneticists to track its movements around the globe in real time. Viruses are best able to evolve as they transmit from one person to another — it is kind of like the telephone game. Mistakes are made as the message is passed down the line of participants.

In a virus' genetic code, the mistakes can be exceedingly small and simple changes like an adenosine changing to a thymine or a guanine to a cytosine. While these genetic code alterations cannot do much on their own to change the way the virus behaves, geneticists can collect many samples and construct a tree of viral descent.

Comparing the genetic code of each person's infection and tracing them back to their sources can reveal how the virus reached its present state, how transmission occurred, and whether the mutations made the virus more deadly. And so, when the virus did mutate around October, the genome platforms were able to identify the new variant accurately and when it first mutated.

April, Friday 13th
Heroism amid depravity

Apart from the first-time ministers, who, for the life of me, I cannot understand why these buffoons cannot use their cell phones to take selfies next to their fancy cars and post them on their Instagram in the quiet of their posh homes. That they are desperate for publicity is obvious. Why use the public broadcaster to advertise their childish antics. I cannot understand. Do they think we are not enough with their snobbishness? Apart from a few depraved cops that behaved like drunks, and the war-starved solders acting like jackasses in public. The blemishes on the sacrifices we the masses were asked to make for one another by the president was cancelled by the flip-flopping of these wayward characters. Apart from these unfortunate instances, all is well.

Amid a contagion, most of us understood that during a complex epidemiological disaster, we needed to suspend the individualistic colonial creed of being anti-authority for once and do what we are told by the president. To act as if one was self-sufficient is delusional, we needed to think of the community first over individualism. After all, does the president not purport to act in our name and in our best interest?

The economic hardships were real, many could not afford to buy food or pay rent. Four weeks into the lockdown, food riots had begun in parts of the Western Cape. I defaulted on the R4000 monthly contribution at the commune where I was a guest at.

Within four weeks of lockdown television and radio began to flood the airways with requests for donations of food ostensibly aimed at sustaining food banks that support the most vulnerable members of communities–the grannies and orphans. Adverts flooded our communities like fury had descended.

'As we fight the spread of COVID-19, e-media in association with the HCI Foundation is partnering with NGOs to provide food to those who need it most. With the scourge of hunger spreading even wider in our community, with each passing day, desperation is growing. The most vulnerable among us need more than our awareness and concern for them. They need help. Now.' The voice of Sally Burdett, Senior e-News anchor, flighted the advert of HCI Foundation. The foundation is raising money from the eTV viewers to contribute to the Solidarity Fund, ostensibly to feed those going hungry every day.

No Kid Hungry deploys volunteers to ensure access to free meals for children in need, especially with schools closed. Salvation Army ensures people have access to food, shelter, and childcare through its nationwide network. Outreach includes drive-through food pickups, community-based food delivery through canteens, and meals at Salvation Army facilities. It also provides snacks and hydration to first responders.

Then there was Mzwandile Masina, the Mayor of Ekurhuleni announcing on POWERfm that on behalf of generous donors–by this he was referring to ANC donors and party tenderpreneurs that he was personally responsible for receiving and distributing food their parcels at the Springs Fresh Produce Market where he and his team had established a Food Bank. Food distribution was done through Ward-based structures and Faith-Based organisations working in the city. Parcels are distributed to the targeted people in need.' He proudly told POWERfm listeners.

The primary target, the mayor said, was 'the existing Indigent list in the city's database.' He also said he was extending the helping hand to orphanages, old age homes and other residents who have the need. 'No money of CoE was spent in procuring the food bank.' People in distress who needed help with food parcels were asked to call a Customer Care number. No sooner had he finished the interview reports surfaced that food parcels were stolen by those in his team supplying they are not-so needy relatives.

Older people were among the most vulnerable to complications from coronavirus. Feeding schemes with a nationwide network of food banks and food pantries were targeted to speed up the supply. I saw nothing given to the elderly folks in Thembisa or Kempton Park. I knew two elderly homes, I checked in and asked if I could help shop and deliver groceries for them. I am glad I did for that is all they ever received apart from their monthly pension.

My cynicism stemmed from what I knew before. The people who are charged with the responsibility of implementing the COVID-19 special social relief of stress grant as well as food parcels from food banks and other suppliers are not men and women with a heart that put others more needy ahead of themselves but put their families ahead in the queue.

The ship of the state is still crewed largely by the same mutinous buffoons that ditched it into the drain during the Zuma years. Unsurprisingly, given the political paralysis, the Mayor took a few of the less controversial bits of the donation offers, dressed them in spandex and sprinkled some stardust, to trot them around the ring one more time. Wash. Rinse. Repeat. It is the same old flannel recycled over and getting threadbare. I had no hope.

The memory of what happened during the time of Zuma is etched deeply in memory. My fear was not an imagined ethereal in my head but real. Reports of malfeasance surfaced shortly after collection from far and near. Considering the corrupt behaviour of the officials in government, some felt justified to kill those they perceive greedy and self-dealing. This is a perfectly justifiable sentiment in the climate of poverty.

※ ※

We are often inhumane, but thankfully, not all at the same time or to the same extent. We are also often kind, good, caring, hopeful, resourceful, and resilient. This pandemic has brought the best and the worst in us, the good and the ugly of our humanity. Quite an interesting mixture of many things, great and small. The fear that paralysed ordinary men and women in the community was balanced by the courageous few among us evidence of humanity's indomitable spirit. No one who lives through pandemic will ever forget this period. It is impossible to overstate the pain and suffering that people have felt and will continue to feel for years to come.

As the coronavirus pandemic forced cities across South Africa to shut down, essential workers have continued to do their jobs. Their work has exposed not only how deep our lines of dependence are but how the inequities of class, race, and industry dictate who may stay inside and who might have no choice but to venture outdoors.

At the height of the pandemic there were images of the kind of absurdity that borders on the macabre. Images perhaps best kept in museums for future generations to remind themselves of the pain and suffering this generation experienced. I remember watching ANC officials pontificating about the importance of well-behaved citizenry then covering their faces in shame when caught by news reporters lying. I remember seeing the high priests of the party flouting the lockdown rules and then showed us the middle finger, even daring the president to fire them from cabinet if he had the courage to do so.

I saw horrid things happening in Gauteng, even worse beyond its borders. I remember seeing a swathe of faces and names of highly trained specialist doctors, nurses, drivers, cleaners, and porters dedicating their lives in the line of duty so that we may have ours. 34 000 of the frontline men and women contracted the coronavirus, most survived while a few were not so lucky.

These are the heroes to applaud, especially because they sacrificed a lot trying to prevent the spread of COVID-19 demon from person to person, from the hospital wards, care homes and community clinics. When the world eventually declares Pandemic I over, we will have all of them to thank for it.

Amid this mayhem, one thing was highly noticeable, the silence of the manufacturers of miracles. The prophets of the charismatic faith were gone during what arguably was the darkest hour of the nation. Why? Evidence the self-acclaimed miracle-workers were a bunch of fake quacks.

Words are not enough to describe the collective grief the national felt. I remember seeing the killing of the poor and vulnerable by the soldiers. I remember seeing solders raiding a home of Colins Khoza at 5th Avenue in Alexander while Colins was chilling.

with a Castle Lite in his yard. Assaulted and later died. No apology offered by the president or Nosiviwe Nqakula except the usual nonsense 'we are investigating.'

I remember seeing defenceless people ripped apart by bullets in the streets of Cape Town. I remember seeing an overweight policeman arrest a Mme Thabede and another hawker vending Achaar and an assortment of vegetables on the streets of Dobsonville, Soweto. I cannot forget the face of Bulelani Qolani who was thrown out of his Khayelitsha shack while bathing himself. Naked. His home destroyed by the metro police.

I remember reading about Shonisani Lethole 35-years old who was admitted in Thembisa hospital one Sunday evening in June after experiencing breathing problems. His father had first transported him to Kempton Park clinic, where he had to queue for two hours in cold conditions before attending to. He was sent from one room to the next, then transferred to the hospital.

By late Tuesday Shonisani had texted his father to bring him food because for 48 hours he had not eaten anything at the hospital. He died the following morning on Wednesday, probably not from the virus, but other complications not established. At the time of his death, neither his father nor the hospital knew if Shonisani was corona positive.

There was trauma inflicted by the pandemic and then the trauma of indignity. Those who were desperately in need of a ventilator were placed on mattresses on the cold floor because of lack of available beds in the hospitals. People in the Eastern Cape hospitals surrounded by filth and shit inside the wards and along the corridors. Insufficient doctors and nurses (those who dared to soldier on with the work) caring for the ill without full personal protective clothing. On top of that doctors having to deal with the daily horror of telling families that their relatives have died.

I remember seeing Italian army trucks in long formations queuing to remove hundreds of dead bodies from hospital morgues to other regions because Lombardy had run out of space to store corpses. I remember seeing casket with a 62-year-old man dead body abandoned in the middle of a busy intersection in the city centre in a town outside the capital of Bolivia. This was a protest, the cemetery having ran out of graves for burial.

I remember seeing gravediggers in Brazil opening old graves to remove the bones of the long departed. Re-filling them with new internments. The message was loud and clear, 'this place is not a place of honour, no highly esteemed dead is commemorated here, nothing of value is here. What is here was dangerous and repulsive to us?'

I remember seeing the president pained not so much by the news of corruption but embarrassed that people in his corner were getting PPE tender deals under questionable circumstances. The PPE meant for the frontline staff to attend to the sick and dying sold to the highest bidder to buy sports cars and holiday homes.

The president was reluctant to set up the multi-agency investigating force to get to the bottom of the revelations in his government, but all the eyes were on him he had no choice, his hand was forced. Officials employed by his government stealing UIF money meant for the people he quarantined two months earlier, millions stolen from the UIF Fund while families waited for their applications to be finalised. Some have had their salaries cut, colleagues preparing for the inevitable retrenchments. This was a final straw on the hopeless. Anger was visible everywhere.

I had a privilege of seeing a makeshift tent next to a private hospital in the suburbs. Many of the cubicle were empty, the beds made up immaculately behind the plastic glass doors, the monitors polished and gleaming, the yards of wires and tubes neatly coiled and hung.

When I entered inside there were signs of change, even down in the cafeteria where the seating area had been closed down and the salad bar had suddenly atomized into constituent, plastic-wrapped pieces of lettuce and broccoli and cherry tomatoes in pairs. It seemed like something was about to happen altered by that omnipresent anxious tension. Hospitals posted 'no-visitor' policy.

I remember seeing a woman on Facetime at a hospital describing her last interaction to her forty-two-year-old husband, who has been fighting COVID-19. Doctors tell her that, despite their best efforts, his life is coming to an end in minutes. Someone carries the phone into the ward, where he lies semi-conscious, so that she can see and speak to him for the last time.

She thanks him for the years they spent together, for his love texts, for making her coffee, for playing games with her, the laughter they enjoyed together and the lovely holidays that enabled her to see the world. As his pulse weakens, she plays their wedding song. A dead silence alighted upon the room. Everything goes quiet and a long silence punctuates the moment. Unlike how we are born, how we die is a profoundly personal and private moment. She is quiet then a flood of tears envelops her face.

One of the nurses reached over and flipped a toggle switch. The doctor strode from the room and the nurses began methodically packing the medical equipment back. The youngest nurse bowed her head and with utter tenderness, pulled the sheet over the patient's face, then shook her head as an expression of sympathy and of resignation. In that instance, all hope was gone for the man and for those watching over him.

There were no families whispering well wishes or holding the patients' hand. There were no favourite hat, blanket, or sweater on the wall except the ventilator, there's no poster boards filled with family photos from graduations, weddings, and holidays at a time when illness has robbed this man of the ability to speak for himself.

In life and in crisis, we seek rituals of connection, but the method of modern hospitalisation robes us of our dignity. Watching someone suffer alone is its own form of punishment. A hospital ward is a theatre where people are expected to. endure their pain by themselves but donate their courage to everyone else. My paralysis was real.

Working with families teaches you to hope that life reconstitutes on the other side of catastrophe and that people can find joy in living again after coronavirus. You do not have to be in a wheelchair to identify. You already know that sad situations sometimes do not get better. Problems do not always get solved. Our families die, and ultimately death rocks our world and shakes our faith to the very core.

We try to manage, like jugglers spinning plates on long sticks. When we feel utterly overwhelmed, we try soaking in the tub, sweating on the treadmill, splurging on new clothes, or heading to the mountains for the weekend. We smile and say we trust in God, but deep down we know it is a lie we are only trusting that God does not permit another deadlier pandemic on us.

Life begins with tears at birth and ends with tears at death. It is simply a part of what it means to be human. It is a truism that just when we appear to hit the nadir of our suffering; we see that we have woefully miscalculated, as things get much worse.

I understand that the dying process is usually a short period, yet an intensely emotional moment. Some people are fortunate in being able to approach their dying process at peace with themselves and with those they love. But this is not always the case, some are confused, unable to express what they need because they are simply afraid to die.

Even though death has existed for as long as life itself, most people are still uneasy about dying. What coronavirus pandemic showed is that the entire nation is scared stiff about the simple fact of dying. We cannot define death. We cannot provide for it. We can give family members no guidance as to how to handle death because there is not anything available. Others mask it with euphemism as if it were hanging on to a life that mattered, not the orderly passage to death.

Grief is a natural response to losing someone loved. There is no right or wrong way to grieve, and everyone experiences it differently. The important thing is to allow grieving and mourning as much as one need to. Next to illness and injury, grieving is intensely painful; in time these feelings begin to subside as a person adapt to a different way of life. Grief can never be fixed, diminished, or stopped, it is part of one's life story and shapes how one lives the rest of one's life.

Integrated grief means the loss becomes integrated into one's autobiographical memory system. Once an individual's grief has become integrated, they are more easily able to engage in other activities without grief constantly preoccupying their mind. The individual finds a way of staying connected to the deceased without their physical presence haunting them.

Acute grief however is something different, it is a lasting form of grief with complicating features that impede the restructuring process necessary for integrated grief to take place. This term is used when grief is thought to have complications that.

prolong the pain of grief without stopping as it should naturally. Complicated grief can go on for years without the intensity of the experience decreasing. Counselling and Clinical psychologist must be sought at the first site of this stage to help heal the grieving person get his/her life back.

In palliative care, practitioners make an effort to meet people where they are as they reconcile themselves to their final hour and to help them discern what matters most to them and then make the effort to arrange their medical care such that it celebrates their personhood at the end of their lives, regardless of whether those lives can be saved.

There's no formulaic way to meet people where they are in their coping, but I learned not to say certain things, such as 'I know just what you're going through,' or especially, 'everything is going to be okay.' You have to say such a thing only once, never mind whether it's spoken out of hope or experience, to learn how it can make a person feel unheard and unseen in their disorientation and suffering, how it can make them enraged.

Prior to the end state, there are physical changes that occur in the person about to die; skin become paper thin, with dark liver spots appearing on hands, feet, and face. Hair can also thin and the person may shrink in stature. Teeth can discolour or develop dark stains. Their external world begins to diminish until the dying person no longer wants to leave the house or their bed and may not want to talk very much. Their mood, character and behaviour also change.

The person begins to sleep for long periods. This can be distressing for relatives, but it is important to understand that even the mildest physical exertion for someone approaching death can be exhausting, and for the moment all effort is being put into staying alive. The dying person often finds it hard to express what they are feeling. At the point of the last switch, the dying increasingly drift in and out of consciousness and finally flatline permanently.

Some relatives may feel horrified by the person's deterioration and find it spooky to sit with them, others may freely embrace the coming to end of a life they have known for long. Understanding and a willingness to communicate openly and truthfully can go a long way. Saying goodbye in person is especially important to the dying. The act of sharing oneself openly and honestly can be very soothing for the dying. With gentle encouragement and support, anxious relatives can often overcome their alarm and find comfort in having done so.

Rituals concerning what to do after death differs from one family to the next from one culture to the next largely based on custom and historical practise held by the tribe. A burial ceremony however appears to be universally held across cultures. However, there is a difference in mourning the dead, the biggest difference is how they grieve, it is personal and unique for each person.

Readers who have undergone serious medical crises and have been dumped at a hospital will immediately recognise the sense of feeling like a wounded, abandoned animal. This is not the inevitable result of the cultural progress itself; it's manmade, a product of both a culture of mass production and less caring attitude. Disease is never neutral. Treatment never not ideological. Mortality never without its politics. In the final analysis, coronavirus the 21st century illness is a metaphor, as well as a memoir of survival.

The following week I attended a funeral of a relative. As the group of men don head-to-toe protective gear and the lid is removed, workers from the undertaker leaves the family to perform the last ritual. None of the men left behind in the sterile, windowless room had met the deceased in life, none knew his religious convictions, and none have mortuary training. They voluntarily undertake the ceremony pursuant to the African custom.

The corpse is dressed in separate pieces of white linen clothing, including a shirt, pants, and jacket. Th body is then placed back inside the coffin and carried out the hearse waiting outside. The men lift the coffin into the back of a flatbed truck and make the long walk to the Nephew's home where a short ceremony takes place.

Hundred maybe two hundred came to his funeral, and fittingly there were several events to mark his passing. One such event his friend stood up to speak. For a few minutes he said nothing at all. We allowed the sadness, the grief, to grow into the silence. He held a space for all of us to feel and did not fill an awkward silence with platitudes or his own reminiscences. When he spoke, he came exactly to the point. He told those gathered there on that day about why social activism was important to his friend, and why the deceased had been important to his small circle of friends. He read the mourners.

The small group of mourners left the home for the cemetery. Section G. They pass hundreds of tombstones, passing mounds of dirt piled atop freshly dug graves. Arriving at the open grave where his body will be placed to rest, they disperse in single line as per the rules.

The workers from the undertaker slowly lowered the body to the floor. Masombuka, the pastor of the mourners, is dressed in a cream-colored panama hat and grey suit jacket, opens a prayer book, and begins reciting prayers and close with an unfamiliar benediction:

Remember that we are but dust

Go in peace, rest in peace, and arise to your lot at the end of days

May the omnipresent console you among the other mourners of Zion and Jerusalem

May they blossom forth from the city like grass of the earth

He throws handful of soil into the grave. It lands on my Nephew's coffin with a thump. The family lines behind the pastor where each throws a handful of soil into the grave until the last of the family member has done so. Then, the front bucket of the skid-steer loader, driven by a man in municipal-supplied khaki overalls waste no time to bring his tractor around and scooped large chunks of soil closing the trench. In under ten minutes the grave is closed. Wreaths are laid, mourners dispersing except the mother and I hovering over the fresh smelling soil to say our final goodbyes and to put the grave marker as a temporary headstone. No one is talking.

A similar scene is the burial of uncollected bodies in City of New York. The sun has barely risen above the glassy surface of Long Island Sound. Already sweating in their hazmat suits, the workers climb 10 ft. up the hole, shovels in their gloved hands. Two coffins are removed from the truck and placed on the front bucket of the skid-steer loader, then driven into the trench where workers pull them off and force them into position, side by side in stacks of three. They fill the spaces between rows with shovelfuls of dirt. Correction officers dressed in crisp navy-blue uniforms stand on the trench's rim, 10 ft. Above the hole. The smell seeps through their protective masks.

A breeze sweeps over an island half a mile from the Bronx where 15 workers watch a backhoe levels the last layer of soil that separates a mass grave from the outside world. There are 1,165 identical pine boxes stacked three high, two wides in this football-field-size pit. The men are here to bury the unclaimed bodies. The backhoe throws a layer of grey sand on top of the soil, making sure boxes are fully covered.

No one knows how many of the people arriving here died of COVID-19. At points, the city was so overwhelmed that bodies were sent to the island before authorities had a chance to determine their cause of death or track down next of kin. Some families chose to have their loved ones buried here. And some families were not aware their relative had died in the first place. 'We figured that most of them would be disinterred because we were moving so quickly,' says the city's department of correction, which oversees operations at the cemetery.

Hart Island is a graveyard of last resort. Since 1869, New York City has owned and operated this potter's field. City workers put unidentified or unclaimed corpses in simple wooden coffins, load them onto a ferry, and entomb them in trenches across the island. The homeless, indigent, and stillborn all lie within eyesight of the hyper-kinetic, high-rolling inhabitants of the Manhattan skyscrapers across the water.

It reflects the lives of people who live on the margins; the homeless, the sickly, the neglected, the forgotten and overworked. Over a century and a half, more than a million people have been buried in unmarked graves on the island, including from past epidemics like tuberculosis, the 1918 flu and AIDS.

I have watched deranged morons telling citizens that this was a 'Chinese/kung fu virus.' The political framing of this pandemic as a Chinese virus needless to say such utterances led to a great deal of stigma around the world for anyone from China (at least for those who believes a moron is an intelligent person, this is normal for them).

I have watched a footage in the BBC showing folks of Chinese descent in UK badly treated by fellow citizens of the UK. The ways in which this pandemic has exacerbated these practices of angry bigots and unhinged evil of American racists is not surprising. It led to violence in the USA, Europe and everywhere outside China. Innocent people squaring up to unbridled bigotry.

I remember reading disinformation from demagogues peddling organics and some other bullshit, telling the world that exposure to sunlight or UVB, hand dryers and injecting disinfectant and bleach would either prevent or cure infections.

※ ※

As well as being a memoir to our survival, coronavirus pandemic is a reminder of how fleeting our time in this earth is. This Japanese term, *mono no aware*, translated roughly 'the pathos of things,' captures a kind of bittersweet melancholy at life's impermanence that additional beauty imparted to cherry blossom human features, as a result of their inevitably fleeting time on earth.

Before now, our levels of happiness were down, understandably so. Rates of suicide and depression soaring is evidence of this. We are not alone many communities in different parts of the world are going through a similar experience. Studies are showing. Many have rushed to blame the lockdown for the isolation we are feeling. We are never short of reasons to justify our irrationality.

Lest we make the same mistake made by others before us, it is worth reminding ourselves that the way to happiness must go through artificial barriers like the lockdown. According to stoicism, a branch of philosophy that came to dominate thinking around happiness in the 1960s. The ideal state of mind is tranquillity, however, not the excitable cheer that positive psychologists usually extoll when talking about happiness.

Tranquillity is achieved not by chasing after enjoyable experiences, but by cultivating a calm indifference towards one's circumstances such as the lockdown we have currently. One way to do this is by turning towards negative emotions and experiences: not shunning them but evaluating them closely instead.

Most of us go through life under the delusion that it is certain events that make us sad, anxious, or fearful. When you hear that a beloved one is ill and feel pained for them, it makes sense to think of the illness as the source of the pain. Look closely at that experience, though, say the Stoics, and you will be forced to conclude that no external event is negative.

Indeed, nothing outside the mind can properly be described as negative or positive at all: what causes suffering are the beliefs you hold about those things. The relative's illness is only bad in view of your belief that it is a good thing for your relatives not to be ill. After all, we know that officially 27000 and counting people died of COVID-19 related illness in the nine months of the lockdown period we hold no beliefs whatsoever about these deaths and consequently do not feel distressed about the numbers.

Stoics often counselled actively dwelling on worst-case scenarios instead staring them in the face. Not only does ceaseless optimism make for a greater shock when things go wrong, and they will. Psychologists have long agreed that one of the greatest enemies of human happiness is hedonic adaptation, which is to say, the frustrating way in which any new source of pleasure we obtain, whether it as small as a new mobile device or as big as overseas holiday, swiftly gets relegated to the backdrop of our lives.

If I ever happened to lose what I had I will not be as devastated because it was never the source of my happiness in the first place. This also includes my attachment to life itself. Being afraid of death led me to hold onto my life with everything I had. Since I released this attachment, joy came with it. While some might feel that thinking about death causes sadness it does give a deeper appreciation and gratitude for the joys, pleasures, and opportunities we all have.

It follows, then, that regularly reminding myself that I might lose any of the things I currently enjoy can reverse the adaptation effect. Thinking about the possibility of experiencing a second and third waves of the virus shifts it from the backdrop of my life back to the forefront, where it delivers a realistic view of life once more.

The second, arguably more powerful benefit of this kind of negative thinking is as an antidote to anxiety. Consider how we normally seek to assuage worries about the future: we seek reassurance, looking to persuade ourselves that everything will be all right in the end. But reassurance is a double-edged sword. In the short term, it can be wonderful, but like all forms of optimism, it requires constant maintenance.

Worse, reassurance can exacerbate anxiety: when you reassure your friend that the worst-case scenario he fears probably will not occur, you inadvertently reinforce his belief that it would be catastrophic if it did. You are tightening the coil of his anxiety, not loosening it.

All too often, things will not turn out for the best. But it is also true that, when they do go wrong, they will almost certainly go less wrong than you feared. Losing your job is unlikely to condemn you to starvation and death; losing a relationship will not condemn you to a life of unrelenting misery. Those fears are based on irrational judgments about the future.

The worst thing about any future event, is usually your exaggerated belief in its horror. Spend time vividly imagining exactly how wrong things could go, you will often turn nebulous fears into finite and manageable ones. Happiness reached via positive thinking is fleeting and brittle; negative visualisation generates a vastly more dependable calm within.

※ ※

Not everything in my observation was bad. Some things were good others utterly admirable, worth telling because they are part of a beautiful human story. I remember witnessing humanity's collective greatness. Individuals reaching out to one another with donations of R5s and R10s and food parcels from their private pantries in an act of solidarity.

I also remember standing to attention saluting a retired 100-year-old English Army Captain, Tom Moore. Tom single-handedly raised upwards of £40million in a month through 100 garden laps in his retirement home all for the NHS frontline workers in UK. Truly, no greater love than this.

Jerusalema is our most popular song released by the rapper Master KG featuring Nomcebo Zikode in 2019. I remember seeing hundreds of posts responding to #JerusalemaChallenge on YouTube. The dance is original from the DRC not South Africa. The world caught on it in a big way and improvised to their liking. Even the president was keen to join in on the action when he challenged his countrymen to mark the South African Heritage Day with their creative moves. Too late Mr. President, the dance had already caught the imagination of the world, well-choreographed on YouTube no improvement necessary.

Jerusalema is not alone but follows on the footsteps of well recognised hymnals. Our national anthem has lyrics conveying a deep sense of trust in God. Its author, Reverend Enoch Sontonga had a revelation of a day such as this when he penned the second stanza, '… God protect her children, save them from destitution and anguish, of diseases and starvation…'

Colourful images of handmade rainbow motifs decorated windows across many cities of the world. Children using a rainbow symbol to remind us they are here, hidden away but hopeful. What is the meaning of a rainbow colour? Rainbows are common meteorological phenomenon seen by every human being since after the floods of Noah. Across the world, cultures have sought diverse meanings in a translucent arc in the sky. However, the hope expressed in a rainbow is frequently tinged with sorrow. But since you can see a rainbow if you are far away from it, and it appears to move as you move, the promise remains elusive.

An idea that thought to have started in Italy; has captured the imagination of the world. Rainbows are a symbol of hope in the world. They appear as perfect arcs, often after a rainstorm when the sun shines into water droplets, shattering its white light into an array of brilliant colours. They are full circles, but to see the half that falls below the horizon, you would have to view the rainbow from above in the sky.

In Christian culture, a rainbow promises better times to come. God sent Noah after the great flood as a sign that people could go forward without fear of another flood. Rainbows are often represented in Western art as a sign of hope and promise of better times to come. In a balcony in Madrid, a banner with a rainbow colours says, 'we will resist.'

Aboriginal peoples of Australia, the rainbow is a very brightly coloured snake that appears to stop their enemies, thought to be the oldest religious belief in the world. In Europe, artists were seen creating portraits of the healthcare workers in the trenches fighting the virus on the frontline. On their canvasses they extolled their virtues, eulogising them as deserving heroes.

Doctors and nurses are treated worse in this country. 'Risk allowance,' or 'special pay' none of this was extended to doctors, nurses, and frontline community volunteers. There were nurses and doctors who completed training but not called to serve the country, instead 200 Cuban doctors were brought in to do what I do not know. When they returned to their country, we were left with a hefty bill.

As a photographic essayist, I documented a better story for our beloved Sons and Daughters of the soil. I created street-level black-and-white digital photo collage layered with 100 video clips. I visited different neighbourhoods and invited passers-by to be filmed and recorded with well-wishing messages for the health givers. Static pictures were replaced by vignettes in a 22-minute video, which stretches across 22.5 metres of giant screen.

I approached the City of Ekurhuleni's department of community development to approve the giant posters to be hung at taxi ranks, shopping malls and in front of hospitals for three months. Request declined citing an obscure by-law regulating the display of adverts. Wow, what a way to show confidence in the citizens!

Bill Gates is no scientist but a philanthropist whose work has been focused on funding research work to find cures to world's infectious diseases. Bill Gates predicted in 2015 probable global catastrophe that would leave tens of millions of people dead. He advised governments to prepare for the spread of a virus created by terrorist for attack, by learning how to make vaccines in a few months the world would be a better place.

'Whether it appears in nature or in the hands of a terrorist, epidemiologists say that an airborne pathogen that spreads rapidly can kill 30 million people in less than a year.' The billionaire told an annual meeting of world diplomats at Davos in 2012. 'And it is quite likely that the world will have to experience such an epidemic in the next 10 to 15 years. No one is listening. We are putting ourselves at risk by ignoring the link between health security and international tensions.'

Bill Gates calls coronavirus pandemic 1, which presupposes a second and a third in the near term. He called on governments to invest in research to develop technologies capable of creating vaccines in a matter of months. Bill Gate's warning was ignored by those who could have acted sooner to prevent the spread of the pandemic.

In a BBC interview in April of the same year of coronavirus, Gates never gloated with self-congratulatory 'I told them so' stance instead, he offered more of his money to fund all promising constructs of coronavirus research, trials and distribution. God multiply this seed!

Thursday, 18th September
From BC to AD

January and February seem like an ancient era–the BC (before coronavirus) compared to the new AD (after domestication). This has been a much more sudden transition than that occurred with the industrial era. This shift will rival great workplace transformations of the 19th century. This pandemic may be the one thing that will finally erase the work and home structures established by the industrial revolution of the 19th century, giving us the opportunity to discover a more flexible, blended approach to navigate the world of work, leisure and home. Starting off their day at home, remote workers are simply not queueing up in the same numbers for a morning venti latte.

For most of us, lockdown and physical distancing have transformed the relationship between work and home, professional life, and family life. It is looking increasingly unlikely that we will ever return to the way things were before.

Let me take the case of Mzwakhe. On March 16th, Mzi left the offices where he worked to head home. That was the last day he assembled with his co-workers in offices redoubt and at the time of writing, no date for return to the office was in site, meaning the new status quo was working better than expected for all parties concerned. No commute time for workers, no rental spaces for tenant employed.

The current shift to AD was enabled by preconditions. First, today broadband services are quick enough to allow for document downloads and video conferencing. We have the advent of 5G connectivity in a way that can enable South Africans to dream differently. Having learned that we can work productively without the daily commute to the office, and that we can convene a meeting over the internet rather than round a table, these habits may persist with benefit to our quality of life and the enviornment. We have social media so people could tell their stories in ways that they could never communicate back then.

Second, advanced economies revolve around services, not manufacturing. Remote work has proven to work and made the new conditions normal again. So, it is going to be difficult to justify returning to the physical environment of bricks and mortar where incurring high rental costs and the headache of commuting under conditions of depressed economy is no longer economically viable.

As a result, the newfound habits working people have developed over the months of the lockdown have the potential to be the basis of our new working reality. We can consciously decide which new habits have served their purpose, which we need to develop and which we want to take into our new reality. It generally takes 12 weeks to form a new habit.

For a change it is in our hands to craft and adapt to a new way of living should we decide. I am excited that we can maximise this opportunity to build a future of well-being for all people and an environment that can sustainably continue to give us abundance of life.

Another aspect of the AD era may be the disappearance of five-day week. In the AD era, the barrier between home and working life will be harder to sustain. The weekend may be lost forever. The rhythm of life has been disrupted and new routines are needed. In a sense, this is a return to a normal only that this is going to be an exciting normal.

Although offices will not disappear, faith in the centralised office may never be restored it is hard to imagine that working life will return to BC ways. Office-dwelling road warriors are now homebound Zoomers, resulting in a bloodbath for airlines, car rentals and hotels. This Zoomification of business meetings is expected to persist for up to two years in the short term.

In a forced makeover, likewise, the cities will have to reimagine themselves as well, with a potential hit of national GDP for the country. Yet, the implosion of the office economy is not necessarily a black-and-white story of ruination. The resilience of cities remains part of the histories of economies.

Wednesday 22nd April
Black Lives Matter

'Brad, you and I have witnessed an unusual phenomenon between 18 million and 28 million people had joined the protests for black lives by the end of July, 2020, and almost half those people were white. Something new is moving in the world. This is a second seismic shift that has happened this year. The death of George Floyd and Jacob Blake in America and the protests that followed it have thrown a spotlight on racism, not only in the USA and Europe but across the world.'

'If one goes by what is happening in the world in the aftermath, the world has a racial reckoning. A shift appeared to have happened with a large cohort of white people, I do not know if this is a 'me too' moment or something that signals a more fundamental shift in human consciousness. Our country's public institutions and communities have fallen under the spotlight for the right reasons. Can you give an opinion as to what caused this shift in consciousness?'

'To be frank, I am not sure why this moment is different from in the past. My response maybe nuanced with personal motives. Donald Trump's demagoguery on race made the problem of American racism legible to whites everywhere in the world in a way that was not there before. Trump's handling of the pandemic response was another major catalyst. As a threat to their own health, for example, and as a disruptor of their own privileged lives. Because of our shared destiny, their response to his conduct has caused us everywhere to examine our individual and collective responses to our local circumstances.

White people in this country have been silent for a long time. I have made this mistake many times. Out of fear of saying the wrong thing or asking an unintentional hurtful question, I tended to not say anything. And the silence is hurtful.

I have always thought that talking about racial reconciliation only makes things worse, believing everything is fine. Some among my friends felt terribly weary and hopeless. I want to give a voice of empathy that communicates that while I may not understand everything; I am willing to walk alongside a brother in pain, rather than immediately moving into a fix-mode. I am willing to learn the pain of racism and prejudice, to learn a language to vocalise, empathise and memorialise pain associated with racial injustice.

This moment made many white people in the world to reflect on their own physical and economic well-being. The lockdown had removed the many of the distractions that in the past allowed us to ignore inequality. I personally felt a physical vulnerability in the face of the virus that made me more empathetic and shifted my priorities to a greater degree. And so, this increased vulnerability has also re-sensitised me towards images of violence against my fellow neighbours, which my privilege had allowed me to tune out to some degree before with justification.

I choose to be outspoken this time around, not because I was pulled along by the current swelling the national mood but because I genuinely felt the pain of others. Now more than before it is feels conspicuous to not change my mind about BLM, not be speaking out or sharing a post or linking to places to donate money and other tangible support for this course. Human dignity is noble.

This new wave of antiracism has created pressure for whites it also created permission for me to express my genuine thoughts. It is now inappropriate for me to be silent in the face of such brutal injustice. I am activated because of my social proximity to Afrikans at work. Look, much of this political foment among us whites happened because of what we see from other white people abroad make no mistake about that. Although much of the conceptual space and groundwork for this moment has been laid there is much conscientizing work that still must happen in my community and among my countrymen.'

Brad and I have not known each other for a long time, the friendship of our fiancés brought us close. Even so, I have no reason to doubt the honesty with which Brad pours out his feelings, and thoughts. In his tone, I do not detect denial, awkward cartwheels and mental acrobatics betraying what he says with his words. In the past it was difficult to engage with the gulf of an emotional disconnect that white people displayed when I articulated my experiences. It was like treacle is poured into their ears, blocking their ear canals. So, it is refreshing for me to hear him speak with this level of candour. But this does nothing to mediate my sunk feelings. I am thinking if it takes an angry, narcissistic, septuagenarian trash like Trump to cause Brad to re-assess his views about me in my own country. This is bad because he is starting from a low base. Trump is a buffoon, a stupid old white man who is trying to be serious but instead is unintentionally funny. Trump's malignant narcissism will grow worse as time goes on. His paranoia will grow worse over time. His disordered thinking will grow worse over time. I must be afraid, very afraid of the white folks in this country if Trump is the yardstick. I surmise that what is changing Brad's attitude is his intense hate for Trump's politics, rather than him seeing me for who I am on my own merit. This causes me to question the place it comes from. It is the saddest moment in our history that white compatriots have given away the agency to be the change they want to see in this country to their elder brothers

> living abroad. There is a part of me that wants Brad his two brothers Matt and Chad to do the heavy lifting themselves before I can accept their bona fides. And I intend to see them to do just that.

This necessitates asking why now, what has changed in the whites' personal lives that moved them off the sidelines into the centre stage bang in the middle of the messiness of life? It was important for me to know how the whites in this country think and feel. In this context, it is opportune to talk about whiteness, privilege, and white supremacy.

Steve Biko once asked who the liberals in South Africa are, he answered the same question thusly. 'It is that curious bunch of non-conformists who explain their participation in negative terms; that bunch of do-gooders that go under all sorts of names. These are the people who argue that they are not responsible for white racism and the country's inhumanity towards Africans.

In short, these are the people who say that they have black souls wrapped in white skins. It is not as if whites can enjoy privilege only when they declare solidarity with the Africans. They are born into privilege and are nourished by and nurtured in the system of white supremacy.'

This list of so-called achievements should be longer and categorically expansive. Better yet? The list should not exist. These firsts are small windows. They are reluctant openings of the narrow avenues to opportunity offered by a predominantly White body of gatekeepers. The homogeneity and decisive power of their institutions are not accidental. They are working exactly as they should.

When you live in a society built on the subjugation of Afrikan lives where Whiteness is the price of entry and anti-Afrikan makes up the totality of its worldview, the collective social and cultural order is not immune to the surrounding context. It draws sustenance from it. Anti-Afrikan thinking is the toxic water in which all creators swim.

White South Africans have always told us that things will be different. For more than 500 years Africans have only had their faith to carry them through the dehumanisation, the broken promise of reconstruction. I can only presume that white people have finally begun grappling with a post-apartheid South Africa untouched by white supremacy that has been defended through privilege, violence, patriarchy, and devaluation of all who are not white.

How I wish all white people could stop to consider the generational trauma of children ripped from their parents' arms, husbands estranged from their wives, fathers separated from their sons and mothers disconnected from daughters. Then, I would tell them, please do not extend your arms marching with us for part of the journey towards decolonisation of this country if you will not pay the full fare.

Please do not extend your hands in camaraderie if you are not strong enough to hear our stories of township life, of many years in shacks squatter camps in the land of our ancestors. Please do not cringe when I ask you, without irony, how many more lives must be sacrificed at the altar of moral conscience.

We need white South Africans of conscience and faith to not only march with us, but also to march with each other in confronting the deprivation and expectation from which they and their forebears reaped reward, whether they are comfortable acknowledging it or not. The urgency of the hour demands nothing less.

I need your kids to ask questions of you and your community about why whiteness connotes purity and goodness in people; why white men are afraid of African men's sexuality, why Afrikans must speak English and minimise their mother tongue, why they must leave in suburbs in order to be accepted by them. The burden of proof must be discharged by those who have historically reaped the spoils associated with whiteness. The dilemma faced by us all should not be a problem for us the Afrikans, rather this is a fundamental barrier that keeps white South Africans from fully realising their humanity with us.

While many businesses will have satisfied themselves with broadcasting messages of support for the black community, others have been waking up to the fact that their policies and inclusion and diversity do not make them non-racist and that Afrikan experience marginalisation as part of their everyday life.

We have always been aware that Afrikans often struggle the most with the burden of shifting identities at work and often struggle to feel as though they can bring their whole selves to the work environment, leading to feelings of being out of place. It is becoming even more obvious that underlying prejudices about cultural difference can influence our perception of a person's abilities and professionalism to the detriment of their career progression.

Brad, as the employer of people have you thought how you might liberate your staff for greater impact in the workplace? How about doing something in your own orbit to make an Afrikan feel seen and valued. This is what it takes to stop racism at company level and for your staff to feel included, valued and affirmed.

Listen – The most important step in the process is to listen to all the voices of colleagues. Let them take ownership of the strategy and give them access to resources and support. Creating safe spaces where staff can share their experiences and concerns and ensuring these are listened to and validated will help you understand their experience and uncover problematic areas and blind spots.

Prioritise reflection – Encourage all staff, especially those who feel they are not directly affected, to learn about and reflect on the effects of systemic racism. Take action that makes it clear this is a priority for your business. For example, Publicis Sapient closed all its offices globally on 19th June 2020 and encouraged staff to observe a global day of reflection in solidarity with the African American community.

Be intersectional – Some companies have traditionally taken a 'one at a time' approach to diversity, which has led to separate initiatives for female, disabled,

LGBTQ+ colleagues. And yet, one employee could encompass all these things. Understanding where experiences intersect as well as where they diverge is vital.

Interrogate your data – While many organisations have been collecting diversity data for a while now, very few of them have visibility of how employee experience, differ by race. In trying to better understand the experience of all staff, many organisations are realising the limitations of generalisation, which blends a diverse array of different groups into one and obscures the systemic racism experienced by individual groups. For example, a strongly represented Asian population may make your organisation look diverse even if there are only a handful of African staff in entry level roles.

Lead by example – If you want staff to prioritise inclusion, then they need to see that it is a priority for you as their leader. From the C-suite down to individual line managers, staff should be able to see that maintaining a non-racist environment where stuff from all backgrounds can thrive is high priority. These small acts of inclusion and overtures of understanding are more apt to cure the racial divide in your organisation than my black anger or your white guilt.'

'For a moment you sound expertly. Did you specialise in diversity studies? Asks Brad.

'Practical experience and life spent inside many organisations with lots of reading.'

'I thought you might find this illuminating extract from an African American writer and activist, Ibram X. Kendi helpful. Kendi reflects an American viewpoint on racism, you might want to balance this view with the classic thought on racism of Robert Sobukwe, the Pan-Afrikan scholar.'

'Given the subtle yet important differences the two writers approach this concept, I think I will be appropriate not rush to discuss this subject right away but give ourselves time to appreciate the differences.' Kendi writes,

One of the most defining questions for Kendi is whether 'discrimination is creating equity or inequity. Kendi's key argument is that there is no such thing as being 'not racist' or 'colour blind' only being actively racist or actively antiracist.

A racist policy is any measure that produces or sustains racial inequity between racial groups. An antiracist policy is any measure that produces or sustains racial equity between racial groups. By policy, I mean written and unwritten laws, rules, procedures, processes, regulations, and guidelines that govern people. There is no such thing as a nonracist or race-neutral policy. Every policy in every institution in every community in every nation is producing or sustaining either racial inequity or equity between racial groups.

Racist policies have been described by other terms: "institutional racism," "structural racism," and "systemic racism," for instance. But those are vaguer terms than "racist policy." When I use them, I find myself having to immediately explain what they mean. "Racist policy" is more tangible and exacting, and more likely to be immediately understood by people, including its victims, who may not have the benefit of extensive fluency in racial terms. "Racist policy" says exactly what the problem is and where the problem is. "Institutional racism" and "structural racism" and "systemic racism" are redundant. Racism itself is institutional, structural, and systemic.

"Racist policy" also cuts to the core of racism better than "racial discrimination," another common phrase. "Racial discrimination" is an immediate and visible manifestation of an underlying racial policy. When someone discriminates against a person in a racial group, they are carrying out a policy or taking advantage of the lack of a protective policy. We all have the power to discriminate. Only an exclusive few have the power to make policy. Focusing on "racial discrimination" takes our eyes off the central agents of racism: racist policy and racist policymakers, or what I call racist power.

The only remedy to racist discrimination is antiracist discrimination. Since the 1960s, racist power has commandeered the term "racial discrimination," transforming the act of discriminating based on race into an inherently racist act. But if racial discrimination is defined as treating, considering, or making a distinction in favour or against an individual based on that person's race, then racial discrimination is not inherently racist. The defining question is whether the discrimination is creating equity or inequity. If discrimination is creating equity, then it is antiracist. If discrimination is creating inequity, then it is racist. Someone reproducing inequity through permanently assisting an overrepresented racial group into wealth and power is entirely different than someone challenging that inequity by temporarily assisting an underrepresented racial group into relative wealth and power until equity is reached.

The only remedy to racist discrimination is antiracist discrimination. The only remedy to past discrimination is present discrimination. The only remedy to present discrimination is future discrimination. As President Lyndon B. Johnson said in 1965, "You do not take a person who, for years, has been hobbled by chains and liberate him, bring him up to the starting line of a race and then say, 'You are free to compete with all the others,' and still justly believe that you have been completely fair." As U.S. Supreme Court Justice Harry Blackmun wrote in 1978, To get beyond racism, we must first take account of race. There is no other way. And to treat some persons equally, we must treat them differently."

The racist champions of racist discrimination engineered to maintain racial inequities before the 1960s are now the racist opponents of antiracist discrimination engineered to dismantle those racial inequities. The most threatening racist movement is not the alt right's unlikely drive for a White ethnostate but the regular American's drive for a "race-neutral" one. The construct of race neutrality actually feeds White nationalist victimhood by positing the notion that any policy protecting or advancing non-White Americans toward equity is "reverse discrimination.

That is how racist power can call affirmative action policies that succeed in reducing racial inequities "race conscious" and standardized tests that produce racial inequities "race neutral." That is how they can blame the behaviour of entire racial groups for the inequities between different racial groups and still say their ideas are "not racist." But there is no such thing as a not-racist idea, only racist ideas, and antiracist ideas.

An antiracist idea is any idea that suggests the racial groups are equals in all their apparent differences.' So, what is a racist idea? A racist idea is any idea that suggests one racial group is inferior or superior to another racial group in any way. Racist ideas argue that the inferiorities and superiorities of racial groups explain racial inequities in society. As Thomas Jefferson suspected a decade after declaring White American independence: "The blacks, whether originally a distinct race, or made distinct by time and circumstances, are inferior to the whites in the endowments both of body and mind.

An antiracist idea is any idea that suggests the racial groups are equals in all their apparent differences—that there is nothing right or wrong with any racial group. Antiracist ideas argue that racist policies are the cause of racial inequities.

Understanding the differences between racist policies and antiracist policies, between racist ideas and antiracist ideas, allows us to return to our fundamental definitions. Racism is a powerful collection of racist policies that lead to racial inequity and are substantiated by racist ideas. Antiracism is a powerful collection of antiracist policies that lead to racial equity and are substantiated by antiracist ideas.

Once we have a solid definition of racism and antiracism, we can start to make sense of the racialized world around us. My maternal grandparents, Mary Ann and Alvin, moved their family to New York City in the 1950s on the final leg of the Great Migration, happy to get their children away from violent Georgia segregationists and the work of picking cotton under the increasingly hot Georgia sun.

To think, they were also moving their family away from the effects of climate change. Do-nothing climate policy is racist policy, since the predominantly non-White global south is being victimized by climate change more than the Whiter global north, even as the Whiter global north is contributing more to its acceleration.

Land is sinking and temperatures are rising from Florida to Bangladesh. Droughts and food scarcity are ravishing bodies in Eastern and Southern Africa, a region already containing 25 percent of the world's malnourished population. Human-made environmental catastrophes disproportionately harming bodies of colour are not unusual; for instance, nearly four thousand U.S. areas—mostly poor and non-White—have higher lead poisoning rates than Flint, Michigan.

I am one generation removed from picking cotton for pocket change under the warming climate in Guyton, outside Savannah. That is where we buried my grandmother in 1993. Memories of her comforting calmness, her dark green thumb, and her large trash bags of Christmas gifts lived on as we drove back to New York from her funeral. The next day, my father ventured up to Flushing, Queens, to see his single mother, also named Mary Ann. She had the clearest dark-brown skin, a smile that hugged you, and a wit that smacked you

When my father opened the door of her apartment, he smelled the fumes coming from the stove she had left on, and some other fumes. His mother nowhere in sight, he rushed down the hallway and into her back bedroom. That is where he found his mother, as if sleeping, but dead. Her struggle with Alzheimer's, a disease more prevalent among African Americans, was over.

There may be no more consequential White privilege than life itself. White lives matter to the tune of 3.5 additional years over Black lives in the United States, which is just the most glaring of a host of health disparities, starting from infancy, where Black infants die at twice the rate of White infants. But at least my grandmothers and I met, we shared, we loved. I never met my paternal grandfather. I never met my maternal grandfather, Alvin, killed by cancer three years before my birth. In the United States, African Americans are 25 percent more likely to die of cancer than Whites. My father survived prostate cancer, which kills twice as many Black men as it does White men. Breast cancer disproportionately kills Black women.

We are surrounded by racial inequity, as visible as the law, as hidden as our private thoughts.' Three million African Americans and four million Latinx secured health insurance through the Affordable Care Act, dropping uninsured rates for both groups to around 11 percent before President Barack Obama left office. But a staggering 28.5 million Americans remained uninsured, a number primed for growth after Congress repealed the individual mandate in 2017. And it is becoming harder for people of colour to vote out of office the politicians crafting these policies designed to shorten their lives.

Racist voting policy has evolved from disenfranchising by Jim Crow voting laws to disenfranchising by mass incarceration and voter-ID laws. Sometimes these efforts are so blatant that they are struck down: North Carolina enacted one of these targeted voter-ID laws, but in July 2016 the Court of Appeals for the Fourth Circuit struck it down, ruling that its various provisions "target African Americans with almost surgical precision." But others have remained and been successful. Wisconsin's strict voter-ID law suppressed approximately two hundred thousand votes—again primarily targeting voters of colour—in the 2016 election. Donald Trump won that critical swing state by 22,748 votes.

The "Racist" and "antiracist" are like peelable name tags that are placed and replaced based on what someone is doing or not doing, supporting, or expressing in each moment. These are not permanent tattoos. No one becomes a racist or antiracist. We can only strive to be one or the other. We can unknowingly strive to be a racist. We can knowingly strive to be an antiracist. Like fighting an addiction, being an antiracist requires persistent self-awareness, constant self-criticism, and regular self-examination.'

Thursday 24th April
A riposte

'I don't remember when my brother and sister became Black. I was 10 months old when my parents brought the six-year-old twins' home. It was not planned or sought out, but my parents were moved to meet them after seeing their photo in the local paper alongside an article about the challenge to find adoptive homes for older Black kids. When my parents discovered that they had already endured three foster homes, they could not say no.

Before I knew colour, before I knew people, before I knew language, before I could do much more than drool, or giggle, or stumble, I knew them. They were part of us. Learning that they were black, and I was white came in bits and pieces and had to be taught. Despite my parents' best attempts at lessons of equality, everything else taught me differently.

My lessons came from watching. I watched white shopkeepers, white family friends, white teachers, white police officers' eye me so differently than they eyed my brother. I watched television shows depict white people as heroes and Black people as criminals, and news highlighting Black crime and minimizing white corruption. I watched trauma — both generational and of his own experiences — trigger rage within my Black brother.

Though I love them as I love myself, bias, prejudice, and racism sunk their insidious hooks into my psyche. I heard too many jokes, slurs, opinions from murmuring white people gathered in circles. I studied their faces as they contorted with mixtures of emotion when I told them I had a Black brother and a Black sister. Hardest of all is that I was not incorruptible. My brother and sister, whom I knew before I knew colour, became Black. And though I love them as I love myself, bias, prejudice, and racism sunk their insidious hooks into my psyche. The carrot of privilege ever dangling in front of me was too much a temptation. I wanted to escape the conflict, move forward, live life, and enjoy it.

Perhaps recapture the memory of a family life before I knew that my brother and sister were Black. That is exactly what I did. As I did so, I loathed the world that made it so easy for me and difficult for others. I loathed myself for choosing to do nothing about it. I am now a pastor for a progressive church in a liberal college town. I was attracted to the openness of the community but noticed that it is significantly less diverse than anywhere I have ever lived. It is an area where it is easy to avoid thinking about racial injustice, because it is not as visible. These facts nagged at me, just as my story has always nagged at me.

I have this life, this story, these things I have witnessed, and emotions I have felt — and I am at a loss of what to do with it all. As a religious leader, people look to me for my opinion. I try to weave my life stories into my sermons but have been reticent to talk about my experiences growing up with a Black sister and Black brother, which is a cornerstone of my identity. I choose not to reveal this too often, because whenever I have, I always felt like I was trying to be the white knight on a black horse.

Using my brother and sister for my benefit, for my defence, for my absolution. But I know that I cannot continue without speaking my truth, no matter the cost. The truth about what I saw and what I see. I am a witness of sorts. A watcher. We are socially awkward neurodiverse autistics are like that. We see it before you do if you ever do. What I saw most from white people, and continue to see, is fear.

By and large, white people are afraid of Black people. As one who has struggled with social anxiety all his life, I know what fear looks like. I saw it in the faces and actions of white kids as we self-segregated on our school campuses. I have seen it in adults and heard it in the way they talk when we discuss racism. Most of all, I know because I had to be taught this fear. It is fear that causes an armed white man to kill an unarmed Black boy. Yes, there is hate, but they hate because we hate anything that we fear.

Even when white people made compromises and gestures of equality, it was always on our terms and by our rules. Maybe it is subconscious for you who claim to have no fear. It is instinctual to fear those who are different. And in that case, one may say that all groups have an instinctual fear of the "other." No shame there. We are a people trying to evolve beyond these instincts, to choose curiosity and commonality rather than hate and tribalism.

But I have also witnessed a different fear and I was never able to articulate it. As I recently marched with my teen son and we chanted "no justice, no peace," it dawned on me. We also fear Black people because we fear justice. In whatever transgenerational memory we have, we know that the reckoning is coming. There has been no real justice. No real reconciliation, or repair, or atonement, or redemption. Centuries of traumatizing and marginalizing people of colour is catching up to us. White people have clutched to power and control as much as Gollum sat in his cave clutching that damn "precious" ring.

Even when we made compromises and gestures of equality, it was always on our terms and by our rules. Real justice is terrifying for the rich and powerful and those complicit in their ways. We hear "defund the police," and how there are much better ways to establish security for society. But security for whom? The police are just a tool. If you want real justice and real change, you need to defund those that use the tools for their control. Justice is scary, because it means making things right and facing one's own complicity in the fact that things are not right.

People are scared to feel the pain caused by their own action and inaction, or the pain of losing anything that relies on racism to survive. In whatever manner that pain may come, deep down we may know it is necessary and inevitable. The thought of racial justice makes many people nervous, but I do not believe we have to be afraid, because there is also something called grace. I do not mean grace from God, but grace from the Black community.

My brother and sister showed us grace as we clumsily navigated being a diverse family. They have shown grace beyond measure. If we really want justice, then we are going to need a lot of grace. We do not deserve it. And we certainly do not deserve it if, after all is said and done, we decide to do what we did almost 200 years ago: give power back to the traitorous, wealthy, land-owning class and give slavery a new name. However, if we repent, truly repent, and let go of what we fearfully clutch, then maybe we can begin again, as family.

Sunday, 26th May
Amanzimtoti

This evening, the president stands ready to deliver yet another speech the nation had been eagerly awaiting. The president gives the weary nation something to look forward to. On Sunday at 20h35 he announces the beginning of easing of the lockdown and the opening of economic activity after 61 days of shutdown. 'We are moving to stage 3,' a confirmation that South Africans would be going back to work kick-starting the comatose economy.

By this time, the president has delivered seven televised addresses to the nation; he sought to bring a measure of calmness to the fraught environment. The nation was both pissed and hungry. This he knew. Understandably. It has been an almost impossibly complicated period for him to navigate since he had no previous reference to fall back on to.

Lockdown could not be sustained, he conceded, however. The timetable he released was confusing, and there was a chart that looked like it had been borrowed from Nando's Peri-ometre. Among the messages he conveyed about staying at home, one crucial subtext was clear: we were now free to drive to our heart's content.

At the crack of dawn on June first, I was in my Honda Civic manoeuvring my way at the Galloyls interchange. Working my way through the morning traffic and at the same time trying to find the right lane amid a convoy of fully loaded horse and trailers is a daunting task. Unwilling to yield an inch of tarmac, their drivers forced me to stay on my lane, honking their horns at the slightest instance of taking a chance in the opening gap that looks apparent between trucks.

In a way, they were telling me my impatience was my problem, not theirs, and I was risking my car at own peril. At this time of the day truckers own the road. All eight may be twelve trucks rumbled on while I was boxed in the middle lane. I could see I was going to miss the one ramp to the N3.

And so, as I was negotiating the end of Bedfordview interchange, I remained extra vigilant because I was fast running out of the tarmac to manoeuvre on. There I was, I missed the onramp and am now driving on M2 to Joburg. *Fuck this, I was not going there.* I stopped, shifted to the emergency shoulder, and reversed the car with the fury of a madwoman. Now, am more than determined to slug it out with the truckers. Fortunately, most had cleared the road by then.

The N3 traffic to Durban slid along with an ease that slowed to a crawl each time approaching the tollgate and would pick up again moments later to a wild chase of other speedsters in my direction. Finally, after four and a half hours on the road, I approached a turn into Panorama Park, a suburb in Amanzimtoti. I headed out on Yellowwood, turning left into Henday, then took the turnoff to Calgary.

I turned off the MP4 player and tuned into radio switching between stations at will. IGAGASIfm found it playing good vibes. The only thing that broke monotony was the radio. Market reports, weather, news, music. It did not matter much which, it was noise and company, and the way things were going I needed both. I played back the VN message sent by Nikki Ayo's friend telling me Ayo is self-isolating straight from work because she has been in encounter with a 'situation.' A relative of COVID-19 patient was not wearing their face mask. 'She is taking this precautionary step to protect all of us.' She added. *very thoughtful*.

I slowed down to take in the view of the suburb, happy to put my woes behind me. I see the city skyline in my rear-view mirror re-appear in front of me again and again. I approached the edge of Panorama Park struck by an unexpected jolt of familiarity at the sight of the sea. From early morning commutes to neon-tinted nights, our streets have become the fabric of our shared history. Whether one live in a crowded city or a deserted outskirt of the town, our streets can tell the story of who we are, where we have been, and where we are going.

A lake came into view below, its waters sparkling in the late afternoon sun. The sweet, refreshing aroma of the surrounding pine forest wafts onto the beach at Lake Forest. Amanzimtoti the sunshine of my heart. As many in parts of the Durban, staycations are popular here this summer, with lockdown putting would-be travellers off venturing too far from home. The hills staggered against each other and tapered down towards the lake surrounding it protectively. Within this expansive nature reserve are vistas of majestic sweep, soaring hills and a hidden gorge. It looked like home. Only more beautiful.

For a large proportion of tourists, Durban south is an experience different to Durban north with its idyllic lakeside break. Around 20% of the property owners own a summer cottage, while more than 50% have access to one via family or friends. Meanwhile there is no lack of beauty spots; two-thirds of the south is covered in forest, parks, and many islands.

While owning a second holiday home is viewed as rather elite in many countries, Durbanites tend not to consider such a privilege, with properties often passed down through generations. A lot of these summer residences are things that perhaps were acquired at reasonable prices. Not every home is equipped to the nines. Many of them are very rustic – you may not have indoor plumbing. While flopping on a lakeside beach might play a role, walks, sport, and DIY are also common pastimes, especially among those bunching together for weeks or more off work.

Ocean View street looked frozen in time, misplaced even as though the quant basket of flowers drooping from the balconies above the strip of shops were forgotten in the years gone by. As I pass by, a woman in a white bonnet waves at me, sweeping the pavement in front of a coffee shop where she worked. I wave with a smile back. The lights in Panorama Park were sparse.

Number 75 is to my right a house standing tall amid other well-designed houses in Richardson street. I swung into the driveway, switched off the engine and pulled the handbrake to the last click. I rested for a short while before opening the door to step into its yard. The weather was unusually warm for the first day of June. I did not even need a shirt. The breeze was growing stronger at 15km/h, and I thought it might be raining later in the evening.

The frangipani trees are not as lush as they have been in summer. Unlike last Sunday when the house was alive with the shrieks of children playing on the lawn, the buzz of the bees around the ixora bushes, the laughter of guests on the balcony upstairs, the clucking of the chickens from the neighbour that sauntered in an out. The yard is silent today.

Ayo's house exudes a quiet peace that envelopes me as I stepped inside.
The entrance to the door was the width of two normal sized doors with elaborate brass hinge. It boasted an opulence that was a beacon for petty thieves. Two stone eagles sat on either side of the door: their mouth open as well as their wide span wings. I stepped inside the hallway and listened intently. It was as if the house which held so many people last Sunday, had shrunk down, pulled into itself. Quiet.

The living room was symmetrical, the couches neatly facing each other across a delicate Queen Anne coffee table, whose legs seemed to barely touch the deep pile of the carpet, wing chairs flanking the fireplace presiding over the room. In the hallway, a chandelier with bulbous crystals hung halfway between the roof and the floor. They sparkled but gave no light. The parquet flooring gleamed, leading further down a passageway into the rest of the house. The stairs lead to the bedrooms upstairs. The stairs curved elegantly in an S shape made stately by their glass-finished balustrade.

I could easily miss the small paint sitting at the corner amid the romp and revelry that surrounds Bacchus, as he leaps from his cheetah-drawn chariot after clapping eyes on the beautiful Ariadne: that tiny detail that transforms Titian's passionate painting of love-at-first sight into something a little less fragrant.

The work, inspired by a scene from Ovid's Metamorphoses, depicts the instant Bacchus's boisterous posse happens upon a heartbroken Ariadne, abandoned by her lover Theseus on the island of Naxos, and has long been cherished for its sensuous portrayal of the way in which the world seems to come to a stop at the moment when people fall for each other.

No sound came from the upper floor of the house. No 'hello, I will be with you just now, now.' Nothing but silence. From the deep shadows at the far end came a sound I knew all too well. Buster flashed across the width of the corridor, his tiny paws skittering on the wood floor as he worked frantically to alter direction. Just before banging into the bedroom doorway, he managed to get himself turned, somehow staying upright on short, splayed limbs. As he caromed off the door frame, he jumped his legs furiously, finally found purchase, and came hurtling down the hallway.

I had just enough time to put down my suite case before Buster was on me, his front paws scrambling at the fabric of my tracksuit and his stub of a tail convulsing wildly. At his full extension Buster barely reached my knees, but his short height did nothing to discourage his enthusiasm. I reached down with both hands and gave the dog an affectionate scratch behind his ears. 'Good to see you buddy.' Then I gently lowered the dog.

Before Buster, Bobo was an extraordinary dog. A big and burly German shepherd, he was as loyal and intelligent as he was frisky and playful. He loved exploring the great outdoors and was a perfect fit for me because I too shared the same love. I used to take him along mountain trailing.

I stepped outside momentarily, the small sett, which doubled as Ayo's outdoor office, was dominated by a large floor-to-ceiling window. In the dusk, the inky blackness beyond would dissolve to reveal an unobstructed view of the ocean. Now however, the window merely framed a reflection of my figure standing in the pool of light from the lamp, my visage staring back at me a reminder of perpetual look of solemnity that never seem to leave me. The reflection looked as tired as I was in person.

High above a solitary mocker poured out his repertoire in blissful unawareness of whose tree he sat in, plunging from the shrill kee, kee of the sunflower bird to the irascible qua-ack of a BluJay. I lingered at the window a little longer. I looked over the sights of figures moving about. The women carrying yokes with buckets of water, of the little *Kinder* scrambling among the carts of goods, the sellers and shoppers, the teenage boys returning from the sports centre.

And then as my eyes floated over the moving figures beneath my window, my gaze fixed on him. Tall, a pointed hat top atop his head, a briefcase in his hand hurrying home. I had seen him several times in the past. How is that I never gave any thought to him or his stature, which seem to have increased in time? And why did my eyes chase over his hasty figure until he disappeared around the corner towards his house? And what was the meaning of that breathlessness rising in my chest and light pinching, that tickling in my belly?

I leaned on the window seal, glanced impatiently at the constant traffic down the busy street, and prepared myself for his reappearance. My eyes fluttered over the.

shoulders steadying yokes and the faces of the Kinder calling each other. There, behind a heavily moving cart laden with used housewares, the pointy hat suddenly overtook the coachman, the buckets and the Kinder. As my heart sang, greeting the hat and the man beneath it, both were already disappearing around the bend out of my sight for good.

I sat there gazing at nothing. Suddenly my mobile vibrates to the sound of incoming VN. My heart-mind flutters at her presence, both near and immediate. In a moment of silence, I seem entirely caught up in an innocuous pontoon full of life and separate from the world around me.

'Hey, hon, someone will be with you just now. Hang tight.' Buster's eyes bright with excitement, the Dachshund stared at me as his tongue lolled out one side of his mouth. Buster stood on his tiny legs that barely kept his low-slung torso off the ground. Not one of the brightest stars in the canine galaxy. He did, however, have a stout heart and a sweet personality.

I retrieved the remainder of my suite cases from the boot of the car one at a time and brought them inside the house and sat by the edge of the couch waiting for 'someone' to appear anytime now. With the last suite case in hand, I activated the car alarm system. Sitting in the lounge felt like I was in a capsule, a gut-wrenching moment. I closed my eyes, wiped away a cold tear and felt a hot one dropping on my cheeks. *I was glad to put the dating game behind me when I met her, the answer to my dreams. Barely twenty days before her birthday. Now this. There are mountains I want to climb and many oceans to sail. There is a world to travel and I do not want to do all this alone If she were to die now, what would my world be without her? The sky would cave in. The boundary walls would crumble and squash the frangipani trees. The Persian rugs on the stretches of gleaming marble floor would shrink. Something would happen. But the only thing that is happening now is my choking, my body is paining from the shaking.*

A feeling of dread washed over me minutes, even hours later with a blur in my eyes. The two worlds, sleeping and waking, that it had been a duty to navigate as a boy has shrunk to a space of a smudge. I waited, my mind light, a weightlessness that moved into my limbs till I felt I might be somewhere in the outer space, buoyant and insignificant.

Restless by the couch, I stood by the hallway, now jittery and anxious, a fresh wind soars, brushing my hair and across my face, pushing a chill down the open neck of my shirt. Outside, the garden is peaceful, undisturbed. The heavy conifer trees sway slowly, while the sagebrush and thistles quiver, bowing before every puff and pocket air. I picture Ayo at the stove, hovering over bran pancakes. I picture myself hunched by the back door in the garden, lacing my steel-toed boots and threading callused hands.

I leaned forward to a sound of a car revving up the driveway followed by beams of light as it came round the corner. I noted a lean man in the driver seat and a woman besides laughing. They parked their car behind mine and the doors slammed, fading as they walked towards the house and then as the doors closed, the sound was swallowed.

A woman walked towards the door opened it and ushered herself inside. She was dressed for a party in short, sequinned dress that shimmered. Her thighs were exposed and the rest of her legs, from the knees down, were clad in tight leather boots. At the sight of me further up the hallway she halts her movement and address me.

'Hey honey, I want you to relax everything is going to be fine, okay. I can imagine you must be tired from the long drive, hungry and worried sick. I am here to take care of things.'

'First, let me take these to your room upstairs.'

'I am boiling water I hear that you love English Breakfast tea.'

'Food delivery will be here shortly, yeah?'

'By the way, I am Nikki, the girl from next door. But for now, I am your welcoming party. Just chill.'

'Nice to meet someone so friendly and welcoming after the intensity of the moment. It felt like eternity standing there by the door.' I say

'I am sure you must have been alarmed to receive a strange message in your mobile hardly six hours after you spoke to Ayo. Kingsway hospital has experienced what they call community transmission the past two days, she has encountered asymptomatic case at the hospital Reception, possibly a relative of a patient in ICU.'

'It's all precautionary, I am sure you know this. I encouraged her to allow me to leave a message on your voicemail so that you are not taken by surprise at the sudden turn of events.'

'She is in her bedroom resting. She will be able to talk when she is up. No doubt, she is upset about this unfortunate turn of events because she had planned a surprising welcome for you including a three-some orgy.'

'Okay, the 'orgy' bit I added it myself.' She giggles.

'I don't know what I am going on about I mean you are the medical expert you should be telling me what to do here.'

Despite Nikki's impishness, my jaws clenched somewhat, lips tightly pursed, eyes darting about saying nothing much by way of conversation. The reality of silence in the house pressed heavily on me. Nikki was still offering me pleasant words flashing me with wrinkles of affection, but I wanted only to evade them. She stood out front, her already slight figure further diminished by a canvass slung over one shoulder failed to inspire confidence.

Nikki is nothing like her best friend–the wild, believes in-fate Ayo. As she leaned into my left side, I caught a waft of her spicy perfume and felt my stomach lurch in excitement. My spirits lifted at the scent. There is calmness in her demeanour though,

Which told me that no matter what happens, she would be able to take care of things. She kept her cool around me, head down, drawing me back to her.

Nikki is upstairs sorting my stuff. I step outside and saunter around the tall palm trees down the unlit pathway in silence. A sense of waiting drifted around me. The bell-shaped yellow fruits hung lazily, drawing buzzing bees that bumped against the window's netting. I felt bereft.

Even now, as I followed a pathway narrowed by shrubs and ferns and darkened by towering fir trees, I felt as if all the intervening years had slipped away, and once again I was retreating into a strange sanctuary. At this time the three-year-old cicadas appears, translucent amber bodies, weightless and eerie, tunnelling out of neat, round holes in the ground to shed their larval shells, sprout wings and fly to tree top, filling the air with the sound of their singular purpose. The male mating song, a vibrating, whooshing, endless hum, a sound at once faraway and up close, makes me feel as though I am living inside a seashell.

The neatly trimmed red beard of Brad, Nikki's boyfriend, is the first to draw my attention. The strong cheekbones, the burning eyes, the smiling lips projecting disarming kindness. A handsome man with warm blue eyes that twinkled with mirth. I was paralyzed. The handsome Brad filling my field of vision and making my insides tremble with a new vibration.

When outside the car Brad extends his warm hand and proceeded to hug me, I hugged him back. His smile reflected on my face, raising a twin smile on my own lips. I stood before him feasting my eyes for a while, straight-backed but breathless and speechless. After a long moment, I bowed slightly.

Brad shoved open the metal door. The air laced with the smell of food came out. Nose poured out like a raucous bird tracing the smell's origin. Brad had brought with him food that Nikki promised me. There was chicken chasseur in one package, a second contained filet mignon, creamed potatoes, and perfectly dressed salmon. A third was a pot filled with pork. The platters are large enough to feed six starving stomachs.

I could not put off examining Brad's expression. He peered up at me to notice that I looked totally astounded. Transfixed. My gaze lowered slightly, and his face relaxed into the most gorgeous smile I have seen.

'Need a hand, Bro?' I asked. He quirked eyebrow up. 'Not really, I'll manage, it's a couple of eats that's all.' 'That one maybe, amended Brad pointing to a package on the floor of the back seat of his expensive looking sedan. I followed his pointed hand still suspended loose in air and saw a larger package covered in silver foil. The red-bearded man smiled at me. Put-off by his slight, I frowned.

He sensed the hint of my contempt. Brad looked up at me, his gaze level. A thin thread of fear spiralled through him when his eyes met mine my narrow eyes almost impaling him. He blinked, staring past me dredging his snappy remark, self-preservation kicked in. 'You cool, Bro?' he wanted to know. 'Yeah, all good.' I lied. 'Cool man.' Easy but weary in his stance.

Brad turned his hair framed his face, and in the glow of the dash, his features were all angles and shadows. He was handsome in a very striking way his confidence had me feel vulnerable. Brad had hard time knowing that my eyes followed him everywhere.

Nikki was well organised, in less than thirty minutes managed to serve us meals. Wine, coffee, and tea sitting on the tabletop. Nikki sets the different platters up and the bowl of fresh salads ready for serving. We briefly debated whether it was a good idea to invite Ayo to the table, after listening to both I persuaded them it was social to dine with her as long as she sits at the far end of the table. She came to join us for dinner.

Nikki settled us around the table, Ayo at the head, Nikki between me and Brad. She captured my hand while Brad held me with one and Ayo the other, we bowed our heads in solemn mode. I felt peace flow through me that was a combination of seeing Ayo and Brad holding my hand as well as the communion of four people united in prayer. Brad's gentle voice and soft-spoken prayer and quiet confidence was the mark of a simple man.

He thanked the Lord for the weather and for work that was done in many parts of the country to help salvage lives from certain death. He thanked God that Ayo was not going to be infected with the coronavirus so that she may continue her mission of administering care to the sick and give hope to the survivors. We all said 'Amen' in unison. My eyes remained closed as a faint remembrance of my own prayers trickling upwards. How long had it been since I felt my prayers were getting through to God? Food was delicious.

'I believe you are married to life-long learning.' Brad teases me

'I am not married to life-long reading. Since you put it like that, I can confirm that I am doing a second Specialisation. I want to heal sick hearts as well as attend to healing the brain too.'

'Seriously?' he protested.

'I spent four years getting my MBA and got away from classes often. I couldn't imagine the discipline required to struggle through Milton on my own.'

'Even if you tried explaining to me what that discipline involves, it will be like instilling in today's teenager an appreciation for Shakespeare and poetry.'

'It is not as complicated as you fear it. In fact, this human organ can be understood completely. The mystery we all want to solve is how the damn thing functions. Everything we do starts and terminates with the mind. Figuring out how the mind functions is what I hope I can do after my research studies, but for now I just want to master the clinical side of the brain fighting the diseases that diminish the brain's computing genius. Hopefully, the next generation of researchers will take the baton forward where we anticipate they will.

Successfully marrying the brain and artificial intelligence into one functioning machinery seamlessly and do something previous scientists have never done. Something awesome.'

All this time Nikki's eyes were trained on me. Ayo's gentle warmth suffusing her cheeks could not stop the smile that curved her lips. The familiar picture, I know. She had dropped her head to the side displaying her best asset. Her unequalled beauty.

'You make it sound easy. Do you mean you can lay it out to me in 8 hours?'

'I can lay it out to you in 10 minutes flat. All of it.'

'And you'll understand everything that happens inside your head. Trust me.'

The brain is the mind, the seat of the soul–the will, consciousness, personality, intelligence, and memory. It is what makes us uniquely human, distinctly apart from other mammalian creatures. This body part has unique special qualities about which a lot must still be discovered by science.

For example, the brain does not feel pain. The brain is not exposed to the outside world, there is no need for it to have pain sensation. You can cut the brain or stimulate it electrically without you feeling any sensation. This explains why we have open surgery, where we keep the patient awake and talking to us throughout the surgery. The brain can remain fully functional for 41 minutes without the oxygen supplied to it before it stops functioning or becomes irreparably damaged. The first guy who worked on the brain gave it the Latin labels we use to describe its functions, which are difficult both to pronounce and remember. Do not worry, the brain does not think in letters only.

The brain is responsible for self-monitoring, organisation awareness, mental flexibility and limiting the behaviour of a person. The four centres of brain, the front, the side, the middle and the back centres perform the higher functions we need to do life. These centres receive and assembles the information we get from outside through the five senses in a meaningful way and stores it magically for future use. The right half of the brain views the left half of the world, and the left half does vice versa.

Intelligence, personality, self-awareness, behaviour, emotions, judgment, problem-solving, concentration, speech, writing, and body movement are controlled by middle side. Understanding a language, memory, hearing, and organisation is processed by the back centre. Interpretation of colour, light and movement are processed by the front centre and words, touch, pain, sensory and visual perception are handled by the side brain.

You cannot tie your shoelaces when a small part called CC is disconnected, it's a bundle of fibres that connects the two cerebral halves of the brain, CC make your hands, legs and eyes to synchronise without this part you cannot do any of this. If the temporal lobe is injured, you cannot identify a person by looking at their face.

My new job after I qualify is to understand the kinds of injuries that happen to the brain as well as the range of diseases that are responsible for handicapping its great functions and find better cure than what exist today. Given the fact that brain is a super computing power, we can laugh at the stupid things humans do and marvelled with awe at the things humans are capable of thinking and bringing into life if given the space to do so.'

Brad and Nikki are kindred spirits. Brad possessed that same zest for life and the ability to make light of any situation. He touted me with the most hilarious queries which kept the night entertaining.

'I had thought I could give you a short ten-minute talk, look at the time now.'

'It was fun giving an unsolicited lecture, you are fun bunch to talk to.'

Although night had arrived, a warm breeze accompanied the tropical climate of the sunshine coast. This weather is different to the chilling Gauteng. Spring had been slow in baring herself. Most of the days are warmish, a sluggard sun making grey mornings and faded out colours on petal flowers come alive. I love how the sounds of ocean waves mixed with starling chimes and rustling fronds.

At 1am, I fell into a dream where it was quiet and everything was misty, could not see my hands in front of me, and walked into a stilted march. Amidst the quiet my footsteps sounded out like a thunder, heavy and booming it frightened me awake. I laid still trying to remember my dream and wondering whether to get up and check on Ayo or camp outside her bedroom as an act of solidarity. *This is going to be one hell of a wait*!

The narrative of our lives sometime seems like a densely woven network of 'not yet now' simultaneously fattened out by the future to which it points, and which, along with the past, makes sense of it. Indeed, it is only because the present is both impregnated and eaten away by a past that makes you someone who waits, and also shapes the future for which you wait, that now is more than an uninhabitable instant.

The question of what to do with the time that is given us in the current moment of the pandemic is certainly pressing, both for those thrust into conditions of impotence and anxious waiting in which there seems to be little to be done, and for those expected to act under conditions of emergency.

But the idea that people understand that the current crisis has somehow released time a time that might be used but that might also be misused is worth attending to. What would it mean to look at the pandemic not just as a public health crisis that requires sound action, but also a crisis of time a moment where questions of temporality and its relation to care have come urgently to the fore?

In waiting, I tried filling time with things I knew well both good and bad. I watched morning shows that were still in season, daytime shows, late night talk shows, soaps, situation comedies, hospital dramas, police series, the drama of Bedford Wives, singing competitions, Australian Master Chef competitions, competitions for business apprenticeships.

Previously flighted soccer games, extreme sports programme, the cavorting of individuals made famous by misfortunes, the fifteen minutes of fame accorded to a young person with large social media following on account of their bizarre act. I watched them all and I hated it.

I hit the remote button, and the television screen shrank and faded into dark picture. I dropped the remote and clasped my hands behind my head leaning back against the headboard, trying to meld my impressions of the stories I have seen.

I no longer have the attention span to watch a show or read a book so I talk to friends past bedtime, the illusion of a schedule at which point I return to Twitter, now slightly unhinged, browse an ex's feed until midnight then shut off the light and hope for the best.

The things that used to keep me alive by which I mean make me feel like a human, with a mind living in a world are gone. The laughter of friends around a dinner table, the buzz of an off-the-cuff flirtation, the high of a long run, the feeling of nailing the arc of an essay, the doing of things.

I pick up the photograph that has been laying on the headboard. Ayo looks about twenty, her mouth twisted in a wry smile, her hair swirling around her face and slender. Ayo is taller than the photo makes her to be a direct contrast to her edges. It did not portray the delicate line of her features, the elusive colour of her long hair, her easy smiles, and the grace in her movements.

From the library shelf, I pulled out a Bible, the Holy Spirit-filled King James version and lay back, flipped it open to the page and tried to meditate on its instructions, then paging through the book of Psalms, I specifically was looking for inspiration, comfort and wisdom. I felt a lift of my heart somewhat, but quickly faded away under the burden of worry. The days floated by, laden with expectation. Days of searching and hope, ending with a void, and then renewed hope for the following day.

To lament the absence of sports seems immaterial at a time when the COVID-19 death toll mounts. What is the point of sport, anyway, when all things are considered? Its theatre and scorelines means little to those who are losing their loved ones, to those fighting on the frontlines. Live sport's absence from the nation's zeitgeist was more conspicuous than most of my favourite obsessions, but its absence was necessary.

Suddenly, standing still and fighting boredom became new sport, along with running a marathon on one's garden. Sport and drama have always been easy bedfellows. For some the very thing that sport gives us, human connection was taken away in an instant when COVID-19 cast its shadow in a doomsday stand-off. Hyperactive people need stimulation, the rest need a distraction.

Those on the fringes of sports industries depend on physical sales to earn a commission selling flags, ice cream, food, beer, and helping customers find parking; the things that make live sports an unforgettable experience. By the end of March the stands fell quiet as food and flag vendors had no customers and hacks tried to reinvent themselves to fill their empty lives. Now there was only one game in the field–the waiting game.

My body flush against the window all day long, looking out to the street. This same window I sat on the first day I came here serves as my link to the outside world one which is increasingly empty and dull.

The reason I sit on this window facing the street is that the street is filled with activities, allowing me to weld those activities into my muffled world. A universe that appears narrowing every day. When I am standing by the window, hands gripping the windowsill I feel connected to the universe again. This gives me time to think while I wait. Ayo has grown accustomed to my obsession and even her demure dog has started hustling me for attention thinking there is something to behold there.

There is a man that lives opposite Ayo's street with whom I have created extant amity. You must wonder what goes through the mind of a man like Uncle Salim. He lives alone; he keeps to himself; his routine is etched in stone. At seven fifteen every morning you see him set out on his jog. Along about ten thirty he slaps the magnetic TECHMAN sign onto the gate of his garage door. The times he leaves his calls vary, but not a day seems to go by without few clients requiring his services either dropping by or asking him for house calls.

Afternoons he can be spotted working around the yard. He will be sweeping the walkway or shaking out the mat or conferring with neighbours on either side. Monday nights, before the trash day, he hauls the garbage bins to the alley. Wednesday nights, the recycling bins. At ten pm or so the three squinty windows behind the foundation plantings go dark.

He is tall, bony man in his late fifties with not-so good posture – head lunging slightly forward, shoulders slightly hunched. Jet-black hair, but when he neglects to shave for a day his whiskers have started coming in grey. Dark eyes, heavy eyebrows, hollows in his cheeks. A clamped looking mouth. Unvarying outfit of jeans and a T-shirt with partially erased looking brown leather jacket when it is cold.

Scuffled brown round-toed shoes that seem humble, like a schoolboy's shoes. Even his running shoes are plain old dirty white sneakers – none of the fluorescent stripes and gel soles and such that most runners wear these days-and his shorts are knee-length denim cut offs.

Uncle Salim has a girlfriend, but they seem to lead separate lives. You see her heading towards his back door now and then with a sack of takeout; you seem them setting forth on a weekend morning in his old VW. He does not appear to have male friends. He is cordial with neighbours but no more than that. They call out a greeting when they meet up with him and he nods amiably and raises a hand often not bothering to speak.

Does he ever stop to consider his life? The meaning of it, the point of it? does it trouble him to think that he will probably spend his next thirty years this way? Nobody knows. And it is almost certain nobody has ever asked Uncle Salim.

On a Monday towards the end of October, he was still eating his cereal breakfast when his first call came in. Usually his morning went; a run, a shower, then tidying up. He hated it when something interrupted the normal progression. He pulled his mobile from his jean and checked the screen, MILDRED.

An old lady: he had dealt with her often enough that her name was in his directory. Old ladies had the easiest problems to fix but the greatest number of crazy questions. They always wanted to know why. 'How come this happened?' they would ask. On the other hand, Mildred was his regular client not the kind you would say his cash cow customer. Although she lived nearby, she often wanted Uncle Salim to come to her.

'Last night when I went to bed my laptop was working fine and this morning it's all kerblooey. But I did not do anything to it, I was asleep.'

'Yeah, well, never mind, I've got it fixed.' He would say.

'But why did it need fixing?'

'That's not the kind of question you would ask about a computer.'

'Why not?'

'Because computers are temperamental things, just like us humans, that's why.'

Another regular client of Uncle Salim is a bowling club member, Barbara has an urgent query regarding her malfunctioning desktop.

'Salim, why I can't seem to get my computer to go anywhere at all, it just completely refuses, it will not go to any website and yet I have a strong Wi-Fi signal in the house.'

'Did you try rebooting it?'

'What's that?'

'Turning off the red button and then on again, like I showed you the last time I was there.'

'You mean sending it off for a time out.' She gave a flutter of a laugh.

'Yes, I did that, but it did not help.'

'Okay, you need to give me twenty minutes and I will be there to check it out, yes?'

'But I wanted to get a present for my granddaughter's birthday on Tuesday, and I need to place the order today for me to get the free delivery when it is ready. Can you come fetch it when I am back?' Uncle Salim stayed quiet, breathing heavy on the mouthpiece.

'Well, she said. Right, 10 am it is then. I will wait for you.

He hung up and took a spoonful of his now cold cereal. He did not like the taste of a cold cereal; he went to warm it in a microwave oven. He finished the last of his cereal and then pushed back his chair. He had a system he set the dishes to soak while he wiped the table and countertop, put away the butter, ran his stick vacuum under his chair in case he had dropped ant crumbs. His actual vacuum day was Friday, but he liked to keep on top of things between times.

His working space was bigger that what you might expect, given that it was in a double garage space. It had a ceiling, two utility shelves on the one side wall for storage of completed work. His toolbox full of state-of-the-art toolkit was sitting on the top shelf. Work bench that was not cluttered with bits of electrical or electronic wires and scrap cut-off parts. The floor was clean laid with vinyl tiles and a carpet piece where he sat on a brown recliner chair. Hanging over his desk was LED lamp. Red.

He closed the garage door promptly at 5:30pm every day, otherwise he closed the main gate leading to the garage when he was away on client visits. He is going to see Mildred now. He paused after he climbed the steps to assess the weather; warmer now than when he had taken his run, and the breeze had died. He had been right not to bother with his jacket. 'Toti has year-round pleasant weather it's surprising to me he would even think of a jacket. He got inside his car, a 1995 Toyota Cressida, started the engine, and raised a hand to Jacobs who was plodding towards his pickup with his lunchbox in hand.

He turns his signal to join the flowing traffic, accelerating towards traffic lights which was amber on approach, slowing his car to an almost undetectable stop. He turned onto Asberry road and parked alongside the curb. But just as he was reaching for his carryall, his mobile rang. He pulled it from his pocket and raised his glasses to his forehead so he could see who is calling. MRS RASHFORD. He punched talk.

'Hello Olivia, what can I do for you this morning?'

'I want to bring my laptop for fixing are you home?'

'I am at a client visit right now, I should be done shortly and will be back by 11h00.'

He stared at the screen a moment before he slid his glasses back and tucked his phone away. The desktop was not much of a repair issue as much as it needed cleaning. But its hardware required attention due to dust and mishandling. After initial inspection, he recommended to take the machine to his workshop to perform a thorough assessment and to a quote for the work to be done. Audrey agreed. Uncle Salim unplugged the computer and loaded it to his Cressida and left. 'I will be in touch.' Cheerio my friend said Olivia.

※ ※

Isolation can become a self-fulfilling prophecy known as the loneliness loop. It can lead to a toxic combination of low self-esteem, hostility, stress, pessimism, and social anxiety, ultimately culminating in the isolated person distancing themselves from others. In a worst-case scenario, loneliness can make people depressed. Support is important during self-isolation. Nikki and I did what we could to keep Ayo from developing ulcers.

Constantly reminding her that she was not alone and that she will pull through this ordeal and emerge the other side in one peace. We encouraged her to spend as much time outside the house, sit outside with a book or clean the house or do laundry, regularly taking the one-hour walk in the street. We encouraged her to go to the local shopping centre once a week to do shopping for food. We cooked meals every day she ate with us at the same table.

Almost the moment that lockdown was announced, I started looking for different recipes for French comfort food desert on Instagram, hoping to spread a bit of sweetness around. I was looking for a nostalgic dessert I could serve that was easy to prepare in advance, something that could add to communal dining.

Rice pudding or *riz au lait* the way French say it. I have a childhood memory of this French dessert and I love it. Nearly every culture around the world has its own version; baked or boiled, spiced, or sweetened with fruit. I cooked the more elaborate version, *riz a l'imperatrice* with candied fruits and alcohol.

When professional chefs put their hand to the dish, however, it is often to add textual contrast. Whenever you are building a dish, you always try to look for different textures, so a bit of crunch. It came to me naturally: crispy, caramelised rice with a touch of fruit. There are recipes that evoke feelings far more than flavour. I found mine.

There is this regressive side to it, where you get to the end of the meal, and the riz au lait comes. The first thing everyone says is, 'Oh, it's way too much. And then it is just like... oh one spoon, two spoons, three spoons...' and suddenly, the bowl is empty. That, to me, is worth all the stars because it means I have served my friends, I have got to the heart of what good food can do to friends, and to pleasure, and to memory.

Last night at the dinner table, Ayo told me about a journal she is developing. She has written down some of her thoughts during her seclusion. I persuaded her that it might be a good idea to share her story with my readers when it is ultimately written.

For the first time I disclosed to her that I was planning to publish a novel on the implications of lockdown. Once the pandemic dust settled, what will people want to read about? History may have answers. In the early weeks, when many people's days were stripped of commutes and school-runs, lunch breaks and gym sessions, it seemed like a good idea to crack on working on a manuscript.

If all the writers started taking notes about coronavirus and handing in their manuscripts simultaneously a year from now, that would be bonanza for the readers. We write for different readership. Literature reflects the diversity of thought and experiences written about. After the pandemic, we are going to have huge reckoning, and literature can help us do that. Reflecting on the COVID-19 and the seismic hold it had clasped on us and how readers batten down the hatches and found another way to process a grief they never knew to expect is an important story to tell.

Fiction helps us process the unique and unprecedented grief; it can help us to feel better. Text variously depict the domesticity, the quiet magnitude of personal loss and the uniquely unpleasant symptoms of our experiences. Escapism may well be another reason, after all, people make art and music to cope with the most extraordinary of circumstances.

Ayo wrote her experience so that she may share the same with those who might be going through similar experience in future pandemics (when she wrote the journal, she had her patients in mind primarily). Not without cajoling she eventually granted her permission to have her story included in my manuscript. Ayo reflects on her feelings and thoughts on waiting and the attendant impact this had on her. Excerpt is an extract.

> Unloading the events of my life onto pages, all sorts of odd fluttering and trickling things that are better left unspoken. Since I woke up this morning the sky is grey, a looming presence unyielding to the sun's intensity. This day is identical to the ones that preceded it.
>
> Over the course of the next two weeks, I am going to trade one life for another, one intimacy for another. There will be no routines dictating my everyday activities, no attachments. Neither a river nor transitory hour can stand still. Trees, suburban silence, green parks, hospital buzz, ornamental plants will not keep me company.
>
> Those of us at home with our commutes on pause, we are realising that bookends to our working day may have served an important purpose after all. The idea of prospection may run even deeper than just thinking about working day. Perhaps the commute also offers an opportunity to tap into deeper levels of creativity, even as we are jostled along a jam-packed traffic.
>
> Reflection is particularly helpful on the evening commute, after the working day is over. And then the mind casts forward to plan the evening, when you come up with a good way of preparing those leftovers. That is the sort of time travelling that happens during boredom and during mind wandering. The third helpful thing about daily commute even if it was for 90 minutes to and fro is resilience. Fighting through the crowds, surviving that little bit of daily drama is missing. Maybe I am mistaking it for habits that I have grown into.
>
> Sitting in an unfamiliar chair, the wood table, my flesh cold, I try to place words on pages, for the first-time words elude me, a confirmation that I was never good with words. Sometimes I know exactly what I want to write but the words refuse to conform to my intentions. Darn it. Maybe I should try another time and a different place for stimulation.
>
> Thinking about stories and trying to get on with writing can often lead to the tricks that the mind loves to play, just to get its own way and keep itself in the world of emotionally exciting thoughts. Proactive thinking helps us avoid becoming wrapped up in an imagined and profitless world of one idea after another. Ideas have a habit of breeding. The mental process of thinking about something interesting or important leads to a flow of ideas that eventually overwhelm my capacity and put me into a sort of dreamy stupor. A place where everything becomes important.

Actions are the only method of reiteration, and it is through reiteration that I finally will reach the perfect idea of how to carry on and work an idea into something valuable. It does not matter if it is writing a story, or starting a business, action is always the most important element for success. Writing a story requires enormous energy the components are manifold and require a juggling act that makes the mind dizzy after a while.

I feel a shiver of apprehension skittering down my neck as if life has caught and dragged me back into its current. My first emotion is not fear but one of anger. I should have known better to take care of myself. Even though my contact with the outside was extremely limited, I encountered asymptomatic people at the reception area of the hospital where I work.

As our street empties of people and ruckus of children, the new garbage appears, clinging to the old garbage, which has become a regular fixture. Dogs burrow through it, especially the piles near the butcher shops and bakeries. Then fear kicks in. The mind will prey on all my insecurities. Am I good enough to do this? Do I fully understand what I am going through? I will be staying awake afraid to sleep in case I might not wake up again.

People hurry home, rushing to beat the dark. People are not silent on the street. When they arrive home, they say a blessing for having held on during the day that had just ended, thanking the Lord for the precious bread he has given them, praying to survive the following day as well. Each person satisfied with their lot and trusting the Lord not to abandon them in their time of need. In my room, I wait for the Lord to answer the same question for *me*.

The sun still hovered over what I could see over the horizon. The day is fading towards oblivion, soon the sky will fill with stars, mother will light the lights and they will have dinner and hurry to bed before the night is over. And the night insinuates its approaching attack of black invites me to play a guessing game from my perch.

Anyone who lives alone has likely wondered and worried at some point how they would get help if something serious happens to them. Although I am a trained physician, somewhere in the middle of my self-isolation, I am beginning to think like normal human beings that I was going to die and even worse; I was going to die alone. Away from the arms of the one I love.

There is a voice of longing inside each woman. We strive so mightily to be good: good partners, daughters, mothers, employees, and friends. We hope all this striving will make us feel alive. Instead, it leaves us feeling weary, stuck, overwhelmed, and underwhelmed. We quickly silence the question, telling ourselves to be grateful for hiding our discontent even to ourselves.

On Tuesday, I was tested. I am waiting with anxiety along with tens of thousands of people just like me whose nose swabs are lucky to be seating at a laboratory somewhere waiting for the PCR machines to prove their innocence or otherwise messiness of life. I have no doubt the thousands of batches have been thrown away into a river somewhere by a lab assistant who feels over-whelmed by the load of work he must process for no thank you from the people he will save with his skills.

COVID-19 turned the fear into a stark and startling reality for me. This epidemic is an isolating illness. Everyone is left to fight it alone to some degree. People in the ICU are never allowed visitors. Doctors and nurses never see them twice, if at all. If you live with other people, you must isolate yourself in a separate bedroom, so you do not give it your loved ones. And when people like me who live alone get it, we must fight the emotional, mental, and physical battle by ourselves. Alone.

I consider myself a professional woman. I have travelled to many countries and take care of myself well. But fighting this illness alone in my apartment is testing me in ways I could have never imagined. It is the hardest, most terrifying experience of my life. Nearer the end of the two weeks, I was afraid to go asleep because I feared I would die in my sleep and never to wake up. Although I do not have symptoms like fever, dizzy spells, shortness of breath, shivers, pneumonia, excessive thirst, nausea, mild pink eye, a rash, lack of appetite, loss of smell, and mounting anxiety. I still do not 'feel fine.'

My body was never weak at the start of isolation or at the end of it, I knew I was still in control 99 % of my usual self, I had the security of knowing someone was on the other side of the door to check on me and ensure I was alive. Here are three things I recommend that helped me triumph over this terrifying illness. I am lucky to have an amazing family two people my fiancé and a friend who has upgraded into a sister both incredible individuals.

I relied on in-person chats with them in ways I could never have imagined before isolating for coronavirus. Video chats became a literal lifeline for me. I love Facetime to bits. I relied heavily on telemedicine with my colleagues who checked in regularly with me as they monitored my progress, telling me if they were seeing changes that would give rise to worry. My sister helped me with breathing exercises through Facetime.

Sharing my experience through Instagram and Facebook was also an extremely beneficial way to feel connected to others. A few days ago, a girl commented that she was in hospital and her dad had just died from COVID-19 and she was really struggling. All I could say was I am so sorry; I hope you are OK. The next day I looked again, about 400 people had engaged with her, listening, and offering comfort. And it meant a great deal to her because they are real people, even though it is cyberspace. Real humans connecting with someone. At the end of day, I am just a woman scribbling away in Amanzimtoti, trying to make sense of things. But that online community has helped me deal with my own experiences of COVID-19 too. There seems to be more openness now. It makes me feel less alone.

Initially I hesitated to do so, but after several encouragement from I am glad my fiancé encouraged me to post my experience, along with my offer to help others with COVID-19, on Facebook. The response, support, suggestions, love, and prayers I got in abundance. This was a gift to me. There is great power in having a community, even at the depths of your weakness. I forced myself to respond to calls and messages. I knew I needed to draw in strength and support from any way I could.

Even if you feel alone, you are not alone. Look around. There are people who want to help you, so say yes when they offer. Or if you need something ask. Sometimes the world seems so dark and lonely, no matter how bright the sun shines or how many people you find within physical vicinity. Sometimes you may feel lost in the world. Sometimes you may feel the world has lost sight of you. But more of us see the light in you than you realize. If we fail to show it to you sometimes maybe it's because we are trapped in the dark trying to get out too. Stay strong, my friends.

There's beauty in the struggle. There's so much to overcome but imagine what it could mean to overcome it. You are truly amazing even if it often goes unseen or unshown. The world only seems so cold and dark sometimes because you are so bright. Your incredible potential sets a high bar.

This one was not hard for me. At my age thirty, I never thought I would come to rely so heavily on my friends. My friend would drop off matzoh ball soup, nutritious meals my fiancé made, Gatorade and fruit, leaving it on the top of worktop in the kitchen.

There is a drawing I did that was *we do not know about tomorrow, but all we need to know is that we love each other*. And for me, that kind of sums it up. We do not know, really. We have got lockdown results but that is all. But ultimately, what gives me hope is the resolve and kindness there is in the community. That is what will win: how we choose to treat each other.

Even though I never felt sick, this virus is incredibly taxing emotionally. Though I have stripped my daily rituals down to their essentials, I remained as scared and as frustratingly human as I was before the world outside screeched to a halt. My friends' efforts kept me alive and literally nursed me to strength.

With constant reminders from my FB friends that 'you are okay, you will get through this and you're stronger than the virus. This taught me a lesson that while I am incredibly blessed to have the kind of support in my life, we have to lean on people who can be positive and give us strength, especially when we don't have it. Our children have better days ahead.

While I was relieved to learn that my second test results were negative and I have been cleared to work again, I am still experiencing the isolation like so many others who live alone. I trust that, in time, this will all be behind us and we will all be able to re-engage with our loved ones as I hope to do.

Defining moments. We all have them. What is important is not the actual moment, really? It is how we respond to the moment that presents. Our own choice. A defining moment is an occurrence or a breakthrough opportunity. Defining moments are a paradox for most of us. This is because they happen all the time, yet most of the time we are unaware. I cannot determine everything that happens to me, but I can define what happens affects me. Our decision to define the moment is what gives us the power to the moment.

I can choose to allow my past to be just what it is; past. The past has already collapsed. A mental construct, one that has been preserved by memories and stories I tell myself. While it has shaped my capsule, the past no longer occupies it. The capsule is an ever-drifting mirage, moving moment by moment across the universe of my life. The present is all I have, and all I ever will.

To be present is to touch and cherish the walls of room no matter how difficult that may be. To let go of yesterday that does not contribute to the beauty of now, to understand that this moment is the only thing that is real in every sense of the word. People in recovery are each looking for something–a shared past, an unexpected future, a place of their own, somewhere to fit in, a lover, a missed mother or father, even just a touch of hope.

I shall take my journal and carefully put it away, blow out the last of the candle, whose wax has coated the candlestick with a colourless film. The streets will become more cheerful, the smells and ugliness evaporate, and this will become the most beautiful place to inhabit. I will be part of it again.

It was Morrison who said, 'We die. That may be the meaning of life. But we do language. That may be the measure of our lives.' The virtue of this life is its being defiantly chosen. Life is to be lived; humanity is won by continuing to play in face of certain defeat. If, in December, we might sing, we need a mother of all parties to the new year.'

Ayo's drama pinpoints with compassion the brutality and insidiousness of the coronavirus pandemic. The narration is disciplined and the sentences plain and sturdy, oars cutting into water, sharp as a blade and laced with uncanny wit. She unpicks the slippery cords of memory and myth that bind mother and daughter, father and son together, hold them apart. Ayo comports herself with gravity and care, the steward of the painful. Her pernickety writing can feel as much ethical as aesthetic.

A harrowing novelisation on another dark aspect of the pandemic. Her telling of the story is subvisceral not detached but restrained. Never didactic but always illuminating even in those dark hours. The ordinary language, the clear pane of her prose, lets her story speak to our heart. This journal is a beautiful, wrenching act of witness, a painful remembrance of an infinite solidarity of humanity - there is a human being in every story of silence. We are called to remember that the past pandemic is never dead. It is not even past, for it lives in our memories.

Her honest, careful words are the equivalent of lightning bolts and thunderclaps. Outside I accept her praise, inside I am flying with the birth of a revelation. It is the first time I realise that there is something I can do to make things different. Not just for me, but for others. This lesson is a piece of gold I will keep tucked in my back pocket for the rest of my life.

We call the months between periods of quarantine the *Hammer* and the period after they produce a vaccine for the *Dance* because it will not be a period during which measures are always the same. Some regions will see outbreaks again, others will not for long periods of time to come. Depending on how cases evolve, we will need to tighten up social distancing measures or we will be able to release the disease again.

There is the rhythm of the dance, the techniques of the dance, and the moves of the dance. It is incumbent on us to learn this new dance as we gear up to adjust to the new way of life. Reading her story made me want to take a stroll through our beautiful parks, to experience the sensation of feet walking down clean sidewalks and paths, eyes taking in the beauty of trees, flowers, and lawns. I will share my deepest secrets and my wild desires with my dearest friend and companion. Ayo.

A fundamental human truth, that, as time passes, things fade, people, relationships, hopes, and dreams fade too. But what transcends are the little daily miracles, illuminations, matches struck unexpectedly in the dark. During this lonely period, I have learned to be responsible to my peers at work and the community I serve as a professional, not to an office full of undisciplined coxcombs.

Right now, most of us are still confined and we must grab small, close utterings of joy to shield our fragile mindsets. Installing bird feeders in our tiny garden ensures a daily offering of winged life. Flitting in and out of each repetitive moment, they have brought such a resurgence of instant happiness. Goldfinches, redpolls, siskins; such glorious names to speak aloud and share simple moments with. In the mornings now, I sit in the garden and watch the birds flying around my new feeders. They are oblivious to all of this. Being able to lose yourself in the world, even just for a bit, is such a crucial part of the journey, I think.

But one thing that has arisen to the top of my list is reading a book in public, something that the president announced we could 'sit in the sun in your local park' had become *verboten*. Because to read in public is to sit down something ascribed to lockdown rules. One of the more unexpected side-effects of lockdown was the innate suspicion and paranoia that had been injected into our daily outings: are we physically distant enough? To be outside now carries an air of performance that might be better expressed as 'Do not mind me, I won't mind you two metres away.

I have a list of books I want to take outside, with a blanket and a bottle of water, and indulge in. A book, then doubles up as the perfect visual indicator that one is taking one's outdoor pursuits under conditions of lockdown responsibly. I might warble that I need an irresistible, joyful, and redemptive book that reminds me of human connection.

A quiet solo activity that might involve sunbathing but is primarily for the intention of reading. Hand signifiers aside, there is such a joy to be found in reading outside especially when we have been blessed with temperate Spring in the paradise of the sunshine coast. A book makes me want to live more attentively. Whenever I pull myself back to the present and the book on my lap, Milton's words echoed my life too closely, its laments of brokenness struck too near my pain.

Hope is such an awkward and personal perception. The emotional response we have to keep going, to find solutions, will vary. Knowing though, that we are all a part of an interconnected ecosystem that miraculously gives light, air, water and sustenance, that has, over billions of years, provided us with everything that is fundamentally necessary to living, provides the brightest form of loving reciprocity. Look up, look out and within. It beats there, hope.

During the lockdown, we have read to transport ourselves to the places beyond our confines. As they lift, we can start to weave those landscapes – the fictional, and the ones outside our front door – together again. I am caressing her cornrows; she likes it when I do that to her. To trace the way strands of hair from different parts of her scalp meshed and held together. Her hair is thick; it always tightened back into a dense bunch right after she ran a comb through it. Trying to comb it now would enrage her.

I suppose it must have started when I was a child, but it came to head at university when it became important to devour books at pace, but with deep focus. And I could only do that one way: laid sprawled on my stomach, perpendicular on the bed, pillows to my right, footboard to my left. The bed had to be made, or it felt weird. I liked the window open. Breeze on the feet. When I am settling into a good book, I do not care if my nook is instagrammable or not, but I care for my back, warmth, and comfort.

I look on people who can read at the kitchen table, on a shaky bus, in a loud and crowded café the same way I do on those who can fall asleep just about anywhere – with colossal, unyielding envy. Me? I need a nook. Ayo's idea of a nook is a front of the apartment or beach with faces onto a busy, sometimes noisy street, car wheels on pavement and bike bells. She tells me 'it all blends together into the hum of a living city that provides what feels more like a sonic backdrop than an interruption.'

As September mixes bouts of glorious sunshine with howling wind and rain, all too often it feels like the unpredictable news agenda is curiously well-matched to the Amanzimtoti spring was like every other I have experienced: stultifying. Relief was sought at the nearby Betsy Pool and the fire hydrants that reckless boys opened with giant wrenches. The cold water made the black asphalt blacker in the black nights. Gossip floated down the street from our neighbour's front verandas and from stoops flanked by big concrete walls.

Nursing a beer, the grownups discussed far-off places. So's son had come back all messed up, and now he was on trazadone. Then the conversation would shift to kids. Sometime the conversation stopped for a moment as girls in summer dresses passed by. Men and women looked at those girls longing, for different reasons, as they ambled down the street pretending to pay no mind to the fine-built boys called to them from a distance.

In short, what I saw in those nights was what our neighbour (uMa) urged me to search for: community. She was a member of the Women's League and had attended the 1956 women's march to Pretoria. When she reminisced about that march, it was with a vividness that made her children feel shy. uMa had been part of community – the burning of the *pass*, boycotts of busses – all these strengthen Ma's conviction that inclusion worked especially if professionals like journalists and sociologists, paid attention to what Afrikan woman built, rather than how she failed.

※※

It is a little over twenty-five weeks, chaos abated. Regrettably, some people never came back from ICU, those surviving hospitalisation continue a long recovery road called long COVID while a majority of people struggle to fill food pantries with basic necessities, unable to pay rent where they live because whatever job they had before has ceased to exist. We will continue to face daunting challenges much of which we were less prepared for.

I was stigmatised by my government, marginalised by my community, and excluded by my neighbour. I was made to feel that I am a foreigner by people who never knew me. I was made to feel the brutality of the police in its raw form. The real-as-hell-feeling I felt there was also a metaphor of a life that has become part of me.

Yet, living here at Toti is different. Serving affluent English-speaking neighbourhood is different. This is what I have always wanted, not living as a white lackey that is, but to be seen, acknowledged, and celebrated for the person I am in the community. I am surrounded by the pace and rhythm of greatness, a place that stops at nothing. I am thorough and incredibly efficient, like an X-ACTO knife. When I see all the endless movement, all the frenzied bustle, I feel alive again. How ironic that I should feel almost like a hero in the eyes of white folks while I am vilified and criminalised by my own.

It is good for now, as I choose to be in the arena. I also choose to live a life that is meaningful not only to me but others as well. Doing the things I want to do, pursuing the goals I want to achieve, and owning every bit of my story. In the start of a new journey, I hope the readers will become my companions along the road.

Saturday, 3rd October
The cost of the lockdown

Outside the driveway we find Brad's dad ready to walk Clara and Click to the park.

'Hello lads,' Nathan greets us proudly, he does care if we respond in time if at all.

'When I was 19, I was already a volunteer for the society for the protection of birds helping the team with land conservation. The Flow is Toti's largest blanket bog, a type of wetland formed from peat. If you have any interest in climate change, restoring and protecting peatland should be close to the top of your list. It is a habitat that is really underrepresented because it's about everything you can't see; what's underneath the surface.'

'A peat is formed when waterlogged layers of sphagnum moss and other vegetation only partially decay, accumulating and sealing in CO_2 that would usually be emitted. These conditions have a cooling effect on the climate by acting as carbon sink. The peatland alone sequesters around 100 million tonnes of carbon.'

'The more you look the more you see' was the maxim I often heard used in relation to the peatland. This is a slow granular world that eventually makes itself known. Its acidic, anaerobic conditions act as a natural preservative, as exhibited by its faithful cataloguing of climatic events across the south of Durban.'

'Among other discoveries, researchers have found fossilised pine stumps dating back to 1100. Prominent features of modernity climate change and population growth mean the proliferation of megacities has widened the risk to our environment.'

'Sage words, Sir. None can disagree with that. The environmental protection is urgent. We cannot afford to postpone our plans not a day more. It is not when but how soon can we do this.' I tell Nathan.

'Okay, I will leave you two to it then. I must walk the dogs and bird watch.'

Following a break, Brad and Nikki are back. Nikki is dying to tell us how their holiday went; so, we paid them a visit in their home. The girls disappear in the kitchen to share photos and catch up on the juicy parts of the holiday experience and update themselves on the neighbourhood gossip. Brad and I could not care two hoots about any of that, we default instead to the usual. Politics.

'Compared with recent past, surely, 2020 must go down as the most dramatic year of this century. I say this with the benefit of hindsight, of course. Do you agree with this characterisation?'

'I would add *defining moment*.' Says Brad.

'What is the one thing shaping the events of this year that stood out for you?'

'Everything that could go wrong in this world has. Less obvious to most people is how this pandemic is the harbinger for the other story that has already been written but has yet to be told. The end of human civilization can be seen in a matter of few decades. The end could come in the form of climate change, mass extinction, ecological disaster, economic depressions, financial implosions, lawlessness, pandemics, plagues, floods, wildfires, and social breakdown. Any of these can precipitate the meltdown.

We are confronted by an unknown virus with no known treatment and without any vaccine or cure we knew we were in bad space. After nine months we had learned a little bit more than we did at start of coronavirus outbreak. Still, we did not know well enough to say we can beat the virus on its tracks. The lowest point of it all was the alarming display of immaturity by world political leaders. We don't know the actual number of people who died from coronavirus, (as of this writing the last report I checked Johns Hopkins University website had estimated that approximately 3m people had died). We don't know what is going to happen to the survivors in the next decade or, what the long-term impact of the virus on the society is. None of us can hazard a guess as to what is coming next.

This year will certainly be part of the storyline where we recount how the coronavirus pandemic swept the world. The swiftness with which it spread, sparing virtually no country, is one of the more astounding aspects of this experience. I should also like to add Black Lives Matter protest at a global scale is a story not likely to be repeated. The phrase topsy-turvy maybe an apt description of the events of this year.

What has happened to us is unprecedented and catastrophic. But in some way, it has been cathartic hastening the passing of the old and forcing all of us to look afresh at other possibilities with a new pair of glasses.

The phenomenon of globalisation is both anathema and a vehicle catalysing change. The collapse of many barriers between nations such as distance, culture, trade, access to markets, commerce, immigration, and political collaboration meant that the world has homogenised into a unified whole. A single village.

The resulting interdependence means a change in circumstances of one nation affects the environment of many nations causally linked to it, where everybody gets affected to a greater or lesser degree by the same thing. We perish together as fools or we thrive as a single humanity. But there is a very real possibility that we could to the extreme end of the spectrum where we disintegrate into closed inward looking nations protecting ourselves against the rest.

First, let me explain the shifting patterns and the impact this has on us. The pandemic has changed our social narrative. The sudden awareness of vulnerability has changed the way in which we think about our health, leisure, and life. This new way of living is described as a dramatic stress test of our individual and collective arrangements and we are discovering the degree to which many of our lives, careers and relationships are precarious.

Another side effect of the pandemic is that is has completely upended what value means in our society. Lockdown has revealed the critical value of low-paid workers, delivery drivers, cleaners, and healthcare workers; social distancing has driven home just how reliant we are on our social and familial structures. At the same time, it has exposed the areas where we have neglected to invest.

Professionals who were once shielded from the effects of economic fragility by comfortable incomes are now finding themselves on furlough with no planned return and experiencing the same uncertainty as those whose finances are characterised by zero-hour work. This seismic shift in self-perception has affected people in different ways.

Now that our established trajectory is in question, we are beginning to reassess what we want our future self to look like. For some, the lockdown has provided a glimpse of a future self with a healthier work-life balance, while others have discovered a desire for fewer financial commitments. For those anticipating a longer, more multi-staged life career, this reassessment can only be a good thing as it will help prepare them for future transactions.

This pandemic has laid bare the shocking inequality that existed before shielded from full view by the steadiness of life. These inequalities are in health, work, and education as well in the extent to which the marginalised groups in the society bear the brunt of this disaster. This realisation has huge implications on our future. While the way in which we will respond to these effects is unclear, what is certain is that they will have a lasting impact on the way in which we live, work and think long after the pandemic subsides.

These inequalities and health disparities are putting poor and most vulnerable in townships, like Thembisa at even greater risk of complications. If by June already patients were made to sleep on the floor and many sat there without food for two days, others dying in hospital make-shift parking lot you must know we have reached a point beyond crisis. The system has collapsed. These are the products of social inequality as much as epidemic dynamics emblematic of the declining social order.

Brad looks at me with a smile. He wags his finger motioning me for the specifics. He wants to know my thoughts not on the performance of the communities but the performance of government in its effort to prevent the spread of the coronavirus and the delicate act of balancing the economy at the same time. He frames his question in neutral tone. Careful not to offend me as an 'immigrant Afrikan.'

> 'I don't want to say we are past the pandemic because we are certainly not, but we are past the lockdown and self-isolation days. Considering all we now know, what are the aspects the government might handle better next time?'
>
> 'I'll tell you what Brad, this is not the right question. At least not for me. I regard myself a radical left and I am angry at the ANC government. My views on the party are considered disrespectful by some and hostile by a few rightfully so. Either way the dice falls, I am indicted. I think nothing of the ANC, I see them as a politically bankrupt beholden to white business captains. They are a bunch of corrupt thieves, like pigs feeding at the trough care nothing for others but themselves. Given this kind of sentiment, do you still think this is a good idea for me to proceed with an assessment?'
>
> 'I do.'
>
> 'You are brave Bro, consider yourself warned.

'Brad, I recognise it is universal among humans to believe in their own fortitude, I get that. But what happens when there is absence of such a belief? Look at us, we lost around 55000 people and counting. The first 15000 casualties up to November is perfectly understandable we did not know enough about the virus to respond effectively, and we did not have the requisite tools to shield ourselves. Those who died in December and later should not have died. Their death was entirely avoidable. In hindsight, the president has one unlucky leader reinforcing the notion Zuma's long shadow hangs like a dark cloud over him. The vaccination programme was simply a nightmare for the president. One faulty step after another. In fact, this is the story of a year you will never want to revisit.

To help remove the notion of escalated bias on my part, let me foreground my thoughts with observations made by political commentators, people who have observed the behaviour of the government and have been interacting with major players in government longer than I have. Mpumelelo Mkhabela, a regular commentator on politics recently wrote an opinion piece in which he expressed the following view.

'A decade ago, when someone asked me if south Africa was at the risk of spiralling out of control and turning into a failed, I dismissed the thought as premature. If I were to return to the same question today and think about what constitute a failed state, my answer would be more considered than dismissive. I still do not think South Africa is a failed state if I consider the definition of the word. The question then arises as to how strong the state in its pursuing its goals.

This is where complication begin to emerge and shows that the answer to the question is neither here nor there. it is also reflected in the state of things in the country over the past decade, which is also neither here nor there. When I travelled through Addis Ababa during the time when there was xenophobic violence in South Africa a couple of years ago, one curious Ethiopian asked me how South Africa is? He was not asking about the weather.

My response was that South Africa is 'so-so.' I could not say that South Africa was unbelievably horrible because that would be gross misrepresentation of the reality. Neither could I say this country is good because that is the sole preserve of the Ambassador. It is his job to tell anyone who cares to listen how great we are as a nation. South Africa has its moments. It has moments of glory in leaders such Luthuli, Sobukwe, Biko, Suzman, Tambo and Mandela. However, this is still the same country that gave us the mutinous buffoon in Jacob Zuma and Cyril Ramaphosa.

A troubling picture emerges when one asks whether South Africa is facing imminent risk of becoming a failed state. It is embarrassing for us as a nation to that at some point in time we had to stop and ask in whose interest is the state power being exercised. The collapse of local government and the dire financial distress that many municipalities find themselves in are not features of a strong coherent state in which citizens can dismiss questions about state failure.

Some would say the problem is not the state, it is only those who steal from it. However, an effective state has at its disposal institutions through which to sanction those that steal from it. If state institutions are experiencing political pushback, when it comes to holding those who steal to account to the public, then a nation has entered a stage of state failure.

The erosion takes place gradually, leading to citizens adapting to living with the rot as they learn to survive under those conditions. South Africans are worryingly becoming accustomed and accepting of living with too many features of a failed state, including lack of safety in their homes and work. It is cause for concern, because at some point it will be impossible to come back from once the country becomes fully-fledged failed state.'

Servaas van der Berg is another social commentator who raised similar concerns in an opinion piece titled *the tentacles of COVID-19 are everywhere* in which he expressed the following view.

'From the perspective of the economy, it has a direct effect on the need to strengthen and expand the health system. But its indirect economic effects are much larger, through the lockdown with all its attendant effects, and the global recession which will continue even after the lockdown is over.

Already, some economists are forecasting a contraction of 10% in economic activity this year, and even this might be optimistic. Economic contractions do not affect everyone equally. Those most affected are tenuously linked to the modern economy. Workers in public employment and in most large firms are relatively protected. The jobs least affected by the lockdown are those that can be done from home using computers and internet connections which favour professionals and skilled workers.

The least protected are those who cannot work from home who have been in low-wage employment, in small firms or engaged in informal activities. Before the crisis, South African income inequality was already extremely high, higher than has been observed anywhere else in the world.

If those losing their income sources were already earning low incomes, this would worsen inequality, but may not increase income inequality all that much. The already massive gap between high income earners and low-income ones will not grow much further when people who had little income to lose become poorer. Thus, measured income inequality may increase moderately from its already exceptionally high level.'

At this point, Ayo and Nikki join us in the lounge finding a muted TV. A sign we are in serious conversation. I felt I have been talking for a long time and was tiring. I could do with their company, may be a change of subject a welcome digression. Ayo winked at me. She was unsure if they should join us to listen in or disrupt the discussion, but Nikki who is tucked next to Brad with her arm around his shoulder is keen to listen. In the end, Ayo the chief host prevailed, deciding it was time to eat. We moved to the dining table where food was ready. A sigh of relief clothed my mood.

Once we had reached the third course. I felt energy restored. Brad had not stopped talking though. His big appetite to engage in politics seems to know no limits. Either he found me garrulous and vain or witty and funny, he was in no mood to share his thoughts about me right now. It was up to me to prove myself that I am not an idiot one way or the other.

'I saw an opinion piece in *The Conversation.*' I continued. 'This article showed that there was a reduction of three-quarters of all informal income due to the lockdown, which would on its own, increase extreme poverty, defined as an income of less than R7000 per person per year, from around 14% of the population to around 21%. But the authors also showed that many informal sector workers were in households where there were also recipients of the child support grant (CSG).

The CSG, the star social policy reform of the post-transition period in South Africa, has been shown to have many benefits, inter alia for child nutrition, stimulating job search and labour force participation of women, and ameliorating rural poverty. Now it offers a vehicle for reaching the poor and enhancing their income at a time when such vehicles are in short supply.

Bassier demonstrated that increasing the value of the CSG would counter the impoverishing effect of the lockdown on informal income. If such an increase in the value of the CSG is large enough, it may even reduce poverty, all other things being equal.

The government to saw the value of using this grant and used it as a major social relief measure, although not quite to the degree these authors had advocated. But the CSG cannot reach all who need social relief. Households fully dependent on informal sector income would not gain from an increase in the CSG and many would sink into extreme poverty, while some who were mainly dependent on the CSG may be lifted above the poverty line.

Other grants have also been increased. The increase in the social old age pension is particularly welcome news for many rural households. Households in rural areas tend to form around income, so the raised old age pension has wide benefits.

The drying up of both informal and much formal sources of income during the current lockdown period changed economic prospects for many South Africans, not only poor ones.

In an economy desperate for sustained long-run growth to lift more people out of poverty, the lockdown and recession will have a devastating effect on small entrepreneurs who must serve as a major engine for growth in any long-run growth process. Economists have speculated that we lost around R1,2 trillion through the lockdown, while the Statistician General confirmed that the economy lost 56% of GDP seasonally adjusted.

> 'The devastation is near total. This means the work of rebuilding the foundations of the economy is going to be monumental.' Interrupts Brad.

> 'Totally.'

The government has touted the introduction of a basic income grant (BIG). Mikhail Moosa examines why the government is considering this grant at this time and why it will fail like all other social experiments in times past. A basic income grant is a cash transfer from the state to citizens to help everyone, regardless of age, employment, or ability, have a minimum level of income. A BIG is likely to be targeted at unemployed people who do not receive a social grant or UIF payment.

This is not a uniquely South African idea. The idea of basic income has a long history and has supporters on both the ideological left and right. Different forms of a BIG have been trialled in Namibia, India and Finland and several trials are ongoing around the world, from California to Kenya. Basic income has recently garnered support in wealthy countries, the UK Labour Party's 2019 manifesto and Spain's recent announcement that it would introduce a similar policy to recover from the coronavirus.

When a BIG was first debated in the early 2000s, economist Michael Samson noted that 'SA's social safety net has a very loose weave.' People older than 18 and younger than 60 falls through the state's safety net. Social grants are designed this way because in theory adults of working age should be able to find jobs, while children and older persons are groups that are perceived to be more deserving of social assistance.

The special COVID-19 grant was supposed to be a temporary remedy, yet millions of applications have been rejected and payments have been delayed. Under lockdown, many people have lost their incomes but still lack state support. A BIG could solve three major issues in the economy.

First, if less conditional, is much simpler to administer than the COVID-19 grant. The latter requires tedious background checks which make the process more cumbersome and expensive. Second, a BIG could put cash in the hands of millions of South Africans who urgently need it. The lockdown has caused an immense economic shock and existing state support is insufficient. Third, a BIG could provide support to millions who fall through the safety net and potentially spur employment. Young South Africans are burdened by exceptionally high levels of unemployment and lack basic financial resources to find jobs.

Based off the minister's comments, it seems unlikely that BIG would be a universal basic income in its true sense. A basic income entails everyone, from billionaires to the destitute, receiving the same amount and wealthier residents pay theirs back in tax. Any potential BIG would not be able to fulfil the loftiest ambitions of a basic income, where the working classes could be liberated from the dull compulsions of economic life and take up more fulfilling and creative labour. A BIG would essentially be an unemployment grant.

Introducing a BIG will be costly. Sceptics sympathetic to the cause of a BIG might argue that the money could be better spent on other welfare policies, such as improving school facilities, creating affordable housing in city centres, or funding social services in townships. A conservative critique might simply reject the principle of the government introducing additional expenditure during an unprecedented economic crisis, particularly when existing funds have not been used optimally.

Basic income is not a silver bullet. It will not heal our divisions or end corruption and it will almost certainly result in tax increases. But social grants have been arguably the most successful development policy under democracy. Grants are not only effective at reaching people most in need and providing income support to poor households, but they also seem to be popular.

A 2018 Afrobarometer survey revealed that most South Africans, across a range of demographics, support providing social grants to the poor. While it is important to scrutinise its affordability, we should also consider whether SA can afford not to provide support to millions of unemployed people. Sceptics should recall perhaps the earliest example of the idea of basic income in Thomas More's Utopia (1516): 'It would be far more to the point to provide everyone with some means of livelihood, so that nobody is under the frightful necessity of becoming first a thief and then a corpse.'

I also came across another article in News24 *Who are the authors of our misfortune*? The author answered that question, 'the ANC.' In its policy conference in 1997, the ANC warned itself through the 'Tactics and Strategy' document where it said there was evidence of leadership in former colonies that had lost touch with their core constituencies. If this were to happen in South Africa, the document said, it had a potential to perpetuate apartheid-era racial, gender and class inequalities.

There was never a choice to have the strong economy in 2020, in any case we were already in a recession by the third quarter of 2019 as you might recall. If people lose income, they stop buying, if they stop buying goods and services businesses die. If businesses die, there is no employment, if there is no employment the depressive cycle accelerate, and it becomes economic depression. The dooms day Sayers are laughing aloud. Because this was taking place contemporaneously with other economies of the world, the world is consequently thrown into deep recession.

The economic cost that has been paid to reduce the infection rate is unprecedented. The drop in employment was faster than anything we have ever experienced before now. Entire sectors of the economy were shut down except agriculture. Every objective marker point to a country unable to live up to its potential increasingly unable to make evidence-based, rational, and morale-building decisions.

This had a degenerative impact on society with inequality rising, unemployment spiking, trust in leaders fell to zero and all-round tension on the rise. Hardship is more widespread, and inequality has widened. Despite the promised support packages, it showed just how inefficient the structures and processes are in getting desperately needed financial support and food to those who needed it the most. It is important to realize that this was not just the result of government policies restricting activities but a series of missteps over an extended time.

These apartheid inequalities would be topped up with a coterie of mainly black men co-opted into the white courtyard of privilege. This would be a potential source of instability and insecurity for all of society, deriving from the same social grievances that underpinned the anti-apartheid struggle. The contributors of this part of the document could not have been more prescient. The ANC, has in many respects, become exactly what the authors clearly warned against: Politically inept and corrupt.

The consequences are exactly as the ANC itself had predicted: Inequalities have not been addressed and a coterie of a politically connected tycoons have joined the white courtyard of privilege. COVID-19 has graphically exposed this reality and more, revealing what statisticians told us many a times about entrenched inequalities. The authors of sections of this document were also correct when they predicted that, if the ANC's behaviour led to the continuation of apartheid inequalities, it would trigger anti-apartheid type of grievances even under democratic rule. Features of these grievances have been in the making for some time now.

And so, when Twitter trended #VoetsekANCVoetsek signalling a stance that [supporters whoever they are] are angry even though they voted for the party at recent elections. Corruption is the signature of South Africa's political class post-democracy. Corruption is woven into the fibre of post-apartheid system. Make no mistake though, action against the corrupt officials in government needs no inter-agency that the president talked of he only meant delays are inevitable. There are enough laws in our book to take the action that is needed.

The state has been instrumentalised to serve whichever political elite takes power. We came together to make a pact about our system of governance–a pact forged from agonising sorrow and suffering and translated in considered reasoning. This pact, our constitution, has never been the destination, it has always been a map of how we get some place better–from a land of deep inequality to a country of peace and prosperity and plenty for everybody.

Corruption always rings heartlessly. But it is hard to understand the type of callousness entailed by corruption relating to the procurement of personal protective clothing. We are not unaccustomed to cruelty and callousness from the ANC; Marikana, Life Esidimeni, the Gupta scandal and everything in between, we have seen it all. The spectacle of corruption when the nation was required to make so much a sacrifice, means we can evaluate the ANC not just as occasional aberration but as always so – our circumstances, however, dire assessed primarily as opportunity for financial gain for themselves, but as always so. Some political commentators have labelled the PPE scandal as murderous. I do not know if there is anyone who can disagree with this view.

It was 11 years of looting of state-owned enterprises, money and general misrules. It was 10 years of populist decisions over prudence. The ANC must understand it does not have the luxury of making grand promises to the electorate because South Africa simply cannot afford it, such politics must change.' The ANC has squandered whatever little opportunity there was to change the lives of the people. Now we are simply 'gatvol with the whole lot.'

※ ※

On balance, the preponderance of evidence delivers a negative verdict. The government did not prepare as well as it should have. When they entered the fray, they executed poorly, saving neither lives nor livelihoods, in the process destroying what little was there in the economy. We have a lived reality, and this is what that reality reflects.

The nation escaped the venomous bite of the virus despite government's pedestrian efforts. I say this Brad, because I am looking at two critical numbers, the rate of recovery as the uncontrollable variable sits at 96%. The death rate, a controllable variable, is sitting at under 2%. The high rate of recovery we experienced was not in the hands of government, i.e. good planning of the public response because they were bad at it. This is attributable to other factors. This, my friend, is God's providence. The hand of God alone shielded us from the devastating impact of the virus.

The UN delegation arrived in the country in September, after they have been here for 30 days, the doctors come out commending the ANC government on its handling of the pandemic. I do not know which Cool Aid they drank, and I do not know why they would play to the gallery. It is a small gallery, and it is of no inconsequence to the people who bore the full brunt of the pandemic and its consequences.

Some among the ANC people would have us believe under the constraining conditions the government's lockdown measures saved us and thus must be grateful. What rubbish! When the pandemic began to spread globally, few governments had the foresight to put together a winning combination of a good preventive plan, the kit those required and the bureaucratic capacity to enact them at scale. To the extent that government's initial efforts were hit and miss, to that extent I will forgive them.

I refuse to credit the government with anything beside. Why? Because they lied the best of times. They lied about preparedness of hospitals, oxygen, testing reagents, PPEs, shortage of nurses and doctors. They lied about buying the vaccines when they were still developed even though South African was a trial site for the J&J and Astra-Zeneca studies.

I reject with contempt any suggestion that the government lived up to its expectations. It never had expectations to begin with because they did not have a baseline against which to measure themselves, and whatever they did they fell below par. The little they did was cancelled out by the scandal of stealing money earmarked to serve the sick and the dying. Excuses are meant to fob off legitimate criticism that must be aired in order for them to acknowledge their shortcomings so that they could do better next time.

Before the pandemic hit, the country was facing its biggest socioeconomic crisis in three decades, extremely high rate of unemployment and a declining investment climate. A broken public health infrastructure, a depleted national fiscus and thoroughly corrupt men and women manning the public service, all of which conspired to make the job of the sitting president worse than his predecessor. The needs of the nation were not the priority of the self-serving cadres who cared rat's ass about service. The frontline staff - doctors, nurses, cleaners had to care for the sick, dying and the hungry by other means.

In one of his addresses the president resigned himself to the fact that 'coronavirus is going to get much worse before it gets better.' Yeah right, Mr president, instead of trying to sound prophetic and clever so late in the day, you should have said that at the start of the lockdown not at its peak. He told a now thoroughly pissed audience that the lockdown had given his government time to prepare the hospitals space to procure equipment and find more beds and to construct field hospitals. What bollocks. Look around.

On this alone, the president lied because three weeks later he was contradicted in the strongest way possible by thousands of nurses refusing to care for the sick at several hospitals due to lack of protective personal clothing at the hospitals. Tender deals relating to the purchase of protective personal clothing were awarded to businesses owned by people and friends in his faction. The focus of investigation by the SIU revealed this much. He was less disappointed by the diversion but pained more by the scandal tarnishing his name. This worried him a lot after all he built his brand around 'Mr clean billionaire.'

Although the nation's initial response was supportive of government's efforts, in the later stages of the lockdown the communities' response varied from lukewarm to indifference. South Africans looked to their government for protection and if those who could afford, to insurers. None came to rescue them.

The government revealed instead a preference to move too fast in the face of imminent risk, but it was forced to backtrack later when mistakes were revealed. Even when foresight's price-tag was small they dilly-dallied. That, in my view was not leading with courage the very thing the president asked the nation to do when he invited the nation to face the pandemic as one. Instead, I saw abdication of responsibility, betrayal of trust and stealing money meant to buy tools to save lives.'

'Very strong sentiments there. Do you have facts to support this assertion?'

'Well Brad, I warned you, didn't I? So, you want facts right? I am happy to let the facts speak for themselves.'

Urban fires were raging wildly in major cities of the world, we know this. I have no doubt we were all aware that the public health care system has been neglected over many decades and was in terrible shape virtually on its knees, hardly in no condition to cope with widespread pandemic conditions. The president was not only faced with an incompetent corrupt bureaucracy he was living in the dark shadow of his predecessor. Nothing he touched ever worked. The vaccine debacle is one sorry example.

By the time government made the decision to lockdown on the 26th March, the first case was confirmed on the 5th at Hiltons, a suburb north of Durban. From the 30th of December to the day of the first confirmed case, government had 90 days. In this time, the government had time to prepare the hospital infrastructure and capacity for the avalanche of cases in the winter months ahead. Our winter proper does not start until late June, early July and it is never cold anyway. Three months is ample time in which to plan and mount a carefully coordinated bold response.

Our only hope was to suppress the coronavirus by depriving the method of its spread, something that was firmly in our hands at individual, family and community level, not the government. When people heard that an infectious disease was spreading widely, some changed their behaviour, avoiding mass gatherings and crowds, others did not care a bit. Ignorance is bliss to the pathogen.

After an initial period of dithering, it surprised me that a full lockdown was announced with such a cavalier attitude. The cost of a hard lockdown was priceless. First, the curtailment of civil liberties for the sake of shielding the elderly was a big ask. We responded by giving without a question. But look at the government ministers – they were taking selfies at their posh houses while eating five course meals, laughing at us the poor. They were flying on a private jet to visit despotic rulers across our borders when fires were burning at home. How insensitive? This is how they have ruled this country for the last 26 years through showmanship–because it was always about them. They dared asking us to do what they were incapable of doing - in private or in public.

Second, by ordering a hard lockdown in March, the government acted too soon, mainly driven by fear. Instead, they should have used the time between January and

April to get all the doctors and nurses at both public and private hospitals ready for the mother of all battles. Secure three month's supply of equipment and protective clothing and then prepare the nation for total shutdown. This would have allowed them time to shut the country down in May through June, at which point the shutdown would have a decisive impact on the spread of coronavirus.

What did they do during the lockdown? Nothing. Instead, they created room for the sceptics to mess up everybody with negativity. The social tools of crowd avoidance, face covering, physical distancing and handwashing on public spaces and especially banning community gatherings of all kinds was never enforced in the way it should have to achieve zero community transmission. The goal suffocating the transmission of the virus, not to inflict pain on us.

The government failed to spot what was coming. When they did, they panicked and acted with childish annoyance. The reported numbers of death and the speed with which those fatalities occurred in China, Italy and Spain left them witless. Consequently, an incoherent response framed much of what was to come as guidance to the public.

South Africa has Embassies, High Commissions and Attaches in many countries including China and Europe. At the very minimum it is expected that the government should have known how many South Africans were doing business in Europe, how many were employed in what part of the world including China between October and January. They should have known those who were travelling to or from Italy, Spain, or Britain, those who were inside the cruise ship that subsequently docked in the port of Durban. That is what governments exist for. Knowing things the rest of us do not and act on the information in their possession to protect their citizens wherever they may be. There is nothing difficult about this its all contained in travel passports and visas.

We are separated by the ocean between ourselves and the place where the epicentre of the epidemic was first identified. In addition, there was a time lag from the first reported case in China and the first case on our soil. All this means the government had enough time to consider empirical datasets, epidemiological modelling and projections thereof including the virus's behaviour in the different settings.

Armed with this of information, there was every opportunity to act with precision because we had time and the experience of the other countries to our benefit. There were ways available to us to block the virus from spreading into this country if this was totally unavoidable at the very least arrest its community transmission. If you include the fact we had the experience of the outbreaks of HIV/Aids, Swine Flu and Bird Flu, the technical knowhow is there. Why on God's earth did we the end up in this sorry state? Lack of knowledge undermined by unpreparedness its undoing.

Brad, in my view, our national response should have been like that of New Zealand. A response that had in its sight the elimination of coronavirus rather than contain and mitigate the breakout. I was already harbouring the fear the government and the public health system were in a horrible shape and they were nowhere near the preparedness levels required for a decisive pandemic response. The president showed once again how weakened the state was. In any case, the supply of protective clothing, the testing reagents and the supply of oxygen was not in the hands of our government but depended on the benevolence of producer nations, who themselves were preoccupied with saving the lives of their citizens.

Acting on real-time information and fact-based science made the difference in keeping the economy going. Taiwan, New Zealand, Japan, Cuba, South Korea, and Vietnam succeeded in this regard. We never had leadership to begin with. The president kowtows to the whims of his faction caring more about what is the correct position to compromise than what was the right thing to do for the poor and helpless.

You want to know what solution I think is possible. You transfer accountability from the state to the individual. How you do this is by causing behaviour change in people through giving them knowledge. This way you lesson fear. You cannot totally eliminate fear in their hearts because we are all dealing with something we don't know but at least it will not immobilise them from acting. The antidote to fear is knowledge. Knowledge is power. This government does not have the capacity to baby seat a nation of 61 million adult citizens. No government does.

By approaching the problem this way the government would have achieved two things; transferring the burden of personal care from the state to the individual and ensuring the consequences of breaching the social rules to eliminate community transmission are borne by the individuals themselves in a way that ensures compliance is sacrosanct. When life and death is in the hands of each person nothing concentrates the mind more.

During the lockdown, the government would have supported the call to action for forty days with real-time data, fact-based information, and science-based advice. Allocating daily three-hour prime time television and radio broadcast to health education specifically information on how coronavirus was behaving to empower the citizens to act with clarity of mind.

Coronavirus is a terrain best understood by infectious diseases community, biotechnologists, virologists, epidemiologists, and data modellers as well as specialist doctors. It is a specialised area one that needed the specialists to be in the forefront of communicating what it is the citizens needed to know to act better in relation to the pandemic. Shining the light on the diseases with actionable information from scientists is a job done by scientists and medical specialists and not politicians.

Believe me, Brad, we would have understood every word the doctors said to us. In instances such as those, the focus on the part of government should have been on building and maintaining a communication infrastructure that reinforce citizen's behaviour change through positive messaging. That is how you battle a pandemic to save lives.

Since the politicians could not dazzle us with brilliance, they baffled us with bullshit served mostly by worst idiots in their rank. We saw them getting bogged down in needless micro-legal tedium, we saw them unable to differentiate meaningfully rules applicable to the different levels of lockdown. The policy controversies and flip-flop on rules blurred the president's labour into a sequence of bite-size comedy. In the end nobody understood the pandemic or why they was shut down.

During this time, the government had known that the number of asymptomatic transmissions of COVID-19, the so-called silent transmissions were high. High viral spread as much as 40% occurred through asymptomatic people. Targeting a specific group of carriers wherever detected, mapping the 'hotspots' and tracking them through was not possible, especially in the rural country like ours. We are a freaking rural country with Gauteng and Western Cape acting as our metros.

With hindsight, we now know that the government's pre-emptive move was never about 'flattening the curve' as they initially claimed rather, they were panicked by the amount of death, which was sudden and unexplained, knowing that the public health system was in the worst shape possible they feared the worst for the country. They thought to themselves if South Africa were to go through a similar experience like that of Italy and Spain, the ANC would find it difficult to explain the deaths of so many folks in one months. That would show at the next polls in the 2021.

Even though the government had assembled the best minds to advise them on the appropriate response to the outbreak, they still panicked in the management thereof. The evidence, over 30000 people died and 51% second quarter contraction in the economy, an approximately R1.1trillion lost in the economy. Add to this over R5 billion set aside for the purchase of PPE ended in the pockets of individuals closest to the president. The net effect is that government succeeded in losing lives and livelihoods.

While there is no denying the threat that Jacob Zuma's faction poses in the ANC, there's also a case to be made that perhaps the biggest threat is those who have the exact same intentions as he did, but are smarter, more tactile, more palatable in the eyes of the donor class, and even more talented at making the message more appealing to the masses. Behind Ramaphosa are men and women ready in the waiting to weaponize everything they have learned from Zuma for their own benefit, and the sooner we accept that reality the more equipped we will be to deal with the ANC weakness.

The idea that we can simply put the Zuma era behind us serves as nothing more than a false counter-narrative to the reality that the mindsets and grievances that brought Zuma to victory in Polokwane will not simply go away once his term had ended. A society where repairs to the government's corrupted past were compromised by a weakened Ramaphosa administration exposed the inherent weakness in the state.

South Africa hardly emerged from an era of total state corruption and sustained economic decline meant state machinery had suffered irreparable damage, its internal organs could not be mobilised to respond timeously with speed. The state had no capacity, it was weak from the inside.

By late May both the Cape colonies had started to climb up the graph in terms of daily infections and total number of deaths per thousand of population, they were far from the peaking point of the infection. The cold winter weather in the month of June made the infections deadly. The Western Cape made great progress by the 10th August infections peaked and death rate slowed to double digits without having suffering enormous damage in capacity loads with minimal dent on local economy.

The Eastern Cape fared badly in comparison, suffering much damage due to strikes and shortage of everything because of endemic corruption in local government. They were overwhelmed by the cases; the army was called in to assist the doctors to cope with the surging numbers of COVID-19 patients.

Indications were that people in the East and Western Cape were simply fatigued by the lockdown. The government had put them in an untenable position where a choice between reducing the spread of transmission by staying at home and starving to death became binary. Rule compliance at level three had for all intents and purposes been rendered academic.

Eliminating the coronavirus was not within government's capability this we knew from the word go. Treating COVID-19 patients meant that the incidence of new cases in defined geographical regions of East and Western Cape and Gauteng could not be reduced to zero in any given time. They hardly had ideas of how to put a descent effort into track, trace, and test. The community transmissions moved quickly from one place to the next, with no one knowing or doing anything about except report post-facto as a statistical fact.

To reduce the rate of infections, the country must have ready the capability of mass testing and efficient contact tracing by the end of April. This they did not have. The next best tool in their arsenal was enforcing a stricter physical distancing at community level. This they did not do. Their lukewarm efforts neither reinforced the rules nor created meaningful awareness on the part of the citizens.

To be successful at knowing where the 'hotspots' were, the scale of testing needed to be at least equivalent to that carried out in Germany at 36 399 tests per day and test results available the same day. But what we saw was testing around five thousand samples a day at the government run labs what was worse their testing machines broke down and the labs ran short of reactive agents. All of this was happening after four months of preparation time and without having reached a peak. Sad.

Far from curtailing the epidemic, the lockdown saw new infections steadily increasing under level five and increased exponentially during the level three, and nothing changed when the country moved to level two. The respite came after we reached the peak in September.

Given the paucity of government data, we have been forced to model the spread of the new coronavirus as if it were a binary phenomenon: individuals are either exposed or unexposed, infected or uninfected, symptomatic patients or asymptomatic carriers. There was no large picture thinking.

Because of lowered resistance to the virus, folks with co-morbidities such as cancer, cardiovascular diseases, hypertension, obesity and type-2 diabetes were faced with odds stacked against them to fight and hold their own against the contagion or face a certain death. This means people from poor communities like the townships including refugees were disadvantaged from the onset.

This is what went wrong with the government's coronavirus response. Government told us to 'stay-at-home, go out only when you buy food, to fetch a grant or see a doctor for something. Go to a funeral of your close relative, not some random folk in the hood when you are out there joining a gathered mass of 50 other folks and keep your distance.' Of course, none of that happened, at least not in the townships. Why, because there was no information given about coronavirus aside from the pamphlets stabled on walls at shopping malls, all of them written in bad English.

Under the conditions of lockdown, it was ill-advised to allow groups of 50 people to gather for funerals when funerals clearly were superspreaders events. In hindsight, it was an error to allow throngs to gather at shopping malls for whatever reason without stringent physical distance enforcement. It was an error to allow the elderly to fetch their pension and other grants in crowded public spaces. This rule had the effect of negating the 'shielding' effect of the lockdown measure we were asked to provide.

By removing super-spreaders events, community transmission goes down. By curtailing the high-risk events like funerals and long queues at shopping centres, the number could have dropped to 1.5 per person. The basics of distancing, masks and handwashing would have been better promoted and if the focus from the start was fighting the spread of the virus socially. The whole regulation process could have been different.

This would have avoided the roast chicken, pyjama, and open shoes fiasco. We fought and squabbled, and even went to courts to dispute minutiae sometime the very existence of the lockdown itself. Meanwhile, infection and mortality were rising. At that time there was still no cure, no vaccine either but that did not mean we should have continued as normal. The fact that government prevaricated so much was more harmful to the quarantined nation.

Hundred and forty-five days after the lockdown, the country moved to level two. At that point we knew more about the coronavirus than we did at the beginning. 145 days later, the relentless Tsunami of infections and deaths never arrived as predicted instead we saw the opposite more patients recovered from the disease after the infection.

There were elementary mistakes that should never have happened. Let me look at some of them. Working against the government's move was the fact they could not quarantine the nation for the second time or ask the nation to give up their freedom once again without a tangible *quid pro quo*. The government did not have a quid pro quo up its sleeves to offer anyone.

If the government attempted to force its way, they would certainly be ignored and kill an already sick economy. My view is, the most reasonable approach, was to invest in prevention rather than treatment approach, with treatment only needed as a fail-safe for cases that fall through the net.

There was this false dichotomy of bringing the pandemic under control and protecting the economy at the same time. My argument is simple the government should have done everything that needed to be done to stop the spread of coronavirus, using every measure at its disposal the economy would recover when the conditions would be more favourable. Biology is biology and it is not interested in what we think. What is more, economy is a human entelechy that can be redefined in countless ways.

Government failed our school-going children because they ignored the advice given. They over-emphasised safety where none applied and excluded other important scientific considerations in the final decisions. By July, the consensus among the scientific community was one that the school-going children were not superspreaders of the virus. In the event they were to be infected at school, they were able to withstand the virus showing only mild to moderate symptoms but never suffering with severe COVID-19 disease. Children accounted for less than 1% of the infections per population. Why stop them?

By all accounts teachers with comorbidities posed a higher risk to everybody, for this reason they should never been allowed to present themselves at schools but shield at home. The drama of courts, demonstrations on the streets for shut down and resistance to the opening of schools was a side show calculated to embarrass the president. But in the main it was fear on both sides that drove the resistance and quiescence. The detractors succeeded in stopping the president from protecting the citizens even with his less than convincing posture.

Soso, a 15 year-old girl, wakes each day before dawn to collect the ingredients her mom needs to prepare vetkoeks which she flogs to the truck drivers passing by at the N3 freeway. Until recently Soso and her little sister spend their days in a crowded mud classroom in Mpophomeni a shack village near Marianhill. When the country locked down to stop the spread of coronavirus their mother, a single parent, lost her job as a domestic worker. She has been out of work since. School remains closed. Even if they were open, Soso could not go back. She is the breadwinner now.

Of the 17 million children forced out of school by the lockdown around the country, 8 million of them are in rural South Africa. Like pupils in rich countries, their education is suffering. But the consequences in poor environments is far worse. In its aftermath, nearly a million children might never return to the classroom, still with nothing to hold onto.

Experts are most worried about the effect on girls. In the handful of places that have reopened schools, such as for example the Ivory Coast, teachers say girls are notably absent. With schools closed, idle girls may strike up a romance or fall prey to sexual predation. Working parents forced to leave their daughters at home all day alone would rather marry them off than risk the shame as consequent to bad behaviour in the form of premarital sex, being raped by relatives or neighbours, pregnancy or experimenting with recreational drugs.

The economic damage from children dropping out of school will be vast. The world Bank estimates that, if schools remain closed for five months, pupils will forgo R10 trillion of future earnings in today's money. That could rise if coronavirus is not curbed and schools stay closed for longer. Thus, the pandemic is widening the pre-existing gap between how much rich and poor children get to improve their chances in life through learning. Unemployment had spiked and the government's promise of food parcels to replace the school feeding scheme had remained just that an empty promise. In this there is nothing ask what is new with this government?

Our government has failed to help children learn from home because of the stranglehold on the access to internet by the mobile phone companies. Due to the problem of high data costs we have low internet access. What the government should have been doing during the lockdown was to call the boards of Vodacom, MTN and Telkom to Pretoria and tell them that in the national interest they must roll out free internet for learners and distribute 4G devises at a subsidised level as part of their solidarity contribution. Period. Radio programming another alternative was easy to reboot during the lockdown. The pandemic gave government an opportunity to press a re-set button and ride the wave to the 4IR digital crest.

As we have seen reopening schools is hard, too. In June only about a third of rural countryside schools said they were ready and had a plan to carry out COVID-19 secure learning and by end of August only 80% were ready. Social distancing is tricky where 40 or 50 kids are often cramped in a single classroom. There were no handwashing facilities in these schools.

School children and their parents lack the political clout of the teacher's union, which typically resists a return to work due to fear of infection. They cite the health risks, which are real. Since schools reopened partially on the 8th of June, nearly 800 schools have had cases reported. Teacher's union SADTU opposed some provinces opening before everyone was ready, demanding that all must hang back. Stupid idea.

When the president announced that public schools will be closed for a period of four weeks and that the 2020 school year will be extended making no mention of private schools, meaning that they can remain open and promote learners to the next grades at the end of the school calendar. Effectively what the president said, there are two systems of education in this country: one for the privileged elites and another for the rest.

This time, however, the right to basic education of those who can afford a private education receives more protection than those who rely on the public system. This is antiquated colonial thinking. There are thus children in public schools with no clear indication of how they will remain on par with their peers in private schools and how this segregated approach will impact on their opportunities for progression and future enrolment into higher education.

Jonathan Jansen pointed out that a massive political standoff would have closed schools, anyway. This way the government seems to be in control. This is a dangerous possibility and not something that should be taken lightly, that government capitulate to the demands of unions at the expense of the children of this country. Ultimately, it seems that a blanket approach was taken because it was easier rather than looking at schools on a case-by-case basis where there was a clear evidence and good reasons to close. This is not just about these four weeks–it is compounded by time already lost and time to be lost in the future if schools close again.

There is nothing inherently wrong with the existence of private schools. But one should not be free while another is bound. I must ask how the politicians and unionists might explain this new tale of two school systems to many other children who challenged similar injustices in 1976.'

Third, the taxi fiasco. The taxi transport business is no more important than any other business in this country, nothing warrants special treatment for the taxi bosses. Like a Bull dog, they are in your face, bark loud, they create an inconvenience but that is what taxi bosses do. After two days, the storm usually dies down and life resumes. As a fact of life, we have learned to live with the taxi nuisance. It's not a big deal.

On the other hand, the taxi bosses had a valid case for challenging the flip-flop stance of government. In April, the government made undertakings to pay special coronavirus relief grants to all kinds of groups, including township businesses. The government knew they never intended to follow through with this promise because they did not have money to fund such extravagance. That in anyone's language is lying.

Here is the irony of it all. The government has set aside circa R10,5 billion to save the SAA airline few people use excerpt themselves when they fly between Pretoria and Cape Town and of their girlfriend/boyfriends with free rides. We know that cumulatively since 2010, the taxpayer has pumped a little over 40 billion into this thing, for what? They refuse to offer the same once-off relief to taxi operators who transports well over 17 million daily commuters. Brad, tell me why is this not duplicity?

At that point almost, all economic activities, two thirds of industries and sectors were on full steam production. Things were substantially looking normal again. Full capacity versus 70% capacity did not make any material difference in so far as the community transmission goes. The question must be asked, why put the taxi operators at such distinct disadvantage if the government did not have a sinister agenda to work them to the ground? Tell me where is equity in government's action in this instance?

Someone must stand up to this corrupt behemoth and tell them, 'go to hell and hang there.' There will be a lot of cheering crowds on the side lines.'

The urge to go for a pee had become urgent by minute. I stood up excused myself and went to the bathroom. Brad used the time to check on his emails, the missed calls and to stretch his legs.

Already without COVID-19, South Africa's economy was in a terrible shape with downgrades, rising public debt (right now debt stands at R4trillion) and devastating unemployment over 50%. Add the four-month lockdown, a global recession it is a desperate picture. COVID-19 was a particularly effective disease at destabilizing public health systems, as well as national economy. What COVID-19 and the impact of the lockdown have done, is to expose the fragility of the South Africa's public institutions. South Africa has been laid bare. The economy will never get back to where it was before. The economic and social consequences of the pandemic have wreaked havoc on our lives and left us all permanently scarred.

All tiers of government can no longer camouflage their mismanagement and terrible performance. Governance fault lines are open. Everybody can now accept that this government clearly lack fit-for-purpose energy much less character.

With foresight and prudent planning, it was perfectly possible to move from level five to opening the economy with a single announcement provided they had the courage to put the foot down on banning all super spreader events, shielding the elderly, the keeping physical distancing and face covering in all public spaces until the end of October, provided further the government insisted on using proven protective technologies that were readily available to the citizens of this country.

Persplex is proven and useful technology and it is cheap. Portable collapsible shields that one erect around one's space including new-look face shields could have played a major role in eliminating the meaningless levels thus saving people needless pain but more importantly saving our economy. There is a disclaimer; all this was possible provided there was a competent public service including civil servants capable of delivering such high demand for services.

In one of his several addresses, the president gave an update on how the government planned to respond to the economic implications of the lockdown. Even as the president announced a set of new measures aimed at saving the economy and countering growing hunger and distress across the country poverty and food insecurity had deepened dramatically just few weeks into lockdown.

The measures would see R500 billion being re-directed in various ways towards relieving those adversely affected by COVID-19. Government said child grant beneficiaries would receive an extra R500 until October, while other grant beneficiaries would get an extra R250 per month over the next six months. Those who are currently unemployed and do not receive social grants or UIF would receive R350 from a special social relief of distress grant.

He announced that a further R 200 billion loan guarantee scheme will be introduced in partnership with banks, National Treasury and the South African Reserve Bank to help companies with operational costs, salaries, rent and supplier payments, among other things. An additional R100 billion will be set aside to protect jobs in the formal economy. Government will also continue to give assistance in the form of loans, grants and debt restructuring to small businesses, spaza shops and informal businesses.

A range of tax relief measures were introduced to lift pressure on businesses and individuals. A four-month contribution holiday was granted for companies' skills development levy, VAT refunds will be fast tracked, and a delay will be granted for the filing and payment of carbon tax.

Businesses will also be given an increase in the turnover threshold for tax deferrals to R 100 million per year, while the proportion of PAYE payments that can be deferred will be increased to 35%. Moreover, no penalties will be applied for late payments if taxpayers can show they were disadvantaged by the coronavirus pandemic. Lastly, taxpayers who donate to the Solidarity Fund will qualify for a tax break.

R162 million from the IDC was approved to support companies for the procurement of personal protective equipment. Calling the scale of the relief programme historic, the president said the government would spare no expense to protect South Africa's people. It was necessary to do whatever it takes to recover from the coronavirus crisis. The president was wrong, that fact proven by his comrades.

On this score, the president was made to look like a fool when undermined by those closest to him inside his party. The predators and the patronage network did not care about the disaster brought by the pandemic, they saw an opportunity for self-enrichment and went for the kill. They calculated where and how much they can take for themselves, considering that rules governing government procurement were relaxed.

They were angry because in earlier years they were prevented from benefitting from government deals by the Zuma faction. This was their time. The predator network immediately circled the state procurement centres eyeing the porous provincial and municipal deals. They scored big time and got away with murder.

The pandemic scrubbed away the polite fiction accepted for far too long; that the ANC government cares. The PPE deals revealed that it was not just Zuma and his people who were the badass crew inside an otherwise morally upright, glorious people's movement. Forget what Ramaphosa says on television, look at the attitude of people around him and watch what they do. It showed us, without a shadow of a doubt, that this party has long been a club of sociopaths.

People who steal our money and food parcels are sociopaths who feel nothing for suffering, or worse, revel in it. People who have a kind of supremacy complex.

People who are only ever calculating how to win in the game, acquire and possess more. People to whom others are meant to end. People who value things over lives.

What happens when you put enough people like that in a government? What happens when a government crosses the threshold into being made of a majority of sociopaths? They have made it normal and desirable even to be selfish, cruel, violent and emotionless, except to fly into rage when all that is questioned. We are considered the strange ones for being disgusted by what is a now openly sociopathic behaviour towards citizens, politics, and economics.

Sociopaths do not have real relationships: our society is just like that, a place of distrust, hostility, and outright enmity. Sociopaths do not consider anyone else a real person, treat them with dignity, respect, care, concern, which is exactly how they treat the rest of us. Sociopaths are narcissists taken to the outermost extreme.

Capitalism tells us that money, sex, power, and fame are all that matter in this life, that acquiring and possessing more of them is the point of life, and the way to get there is to dominate and exploit others. Capitalism has turned them into slaves for another rand, hook up fan, like, follower, even as they dance to the tune of their own self-destruction.

Capitalism is what made them selfish, stupid, brutal, violent because they have been conditioned their whole lives to be consumers but not decent human beings, thoughtful, sane, and kind people. Because the year was so depressing, grim, and relentless was not just the natural calamity. It was this calamity that revealed the truth about us. And that truth is ugly. We are violent, brutal and indifferent nation. There is enough to make our societies that way, period. But the folks working in government added catastrophe to our calamity.

And if you are a sane, decent person standing on the side lines watching well, how do you live in such a place? A dehumanized, violent, brutal country of hungry hyena dogs? How do you live in a society of sociopaths? Isn't it an oxymoron to begin with? Where do you go from there? How do you coexist with the kind of remorseless people who do not care about causing death on this scale? How do you not shudder in contempt and disgrace every time you see them which is all the time? But where does that leave you?

That is my question to you. The pandemic revealed that our country has a total lack of empathy, goodness, decency but a stunning capacity for indifference, malice, carelessness, selfishness and violence.

The tools at the disposal of the government to assist were limited and difficult to use: the scope of mismanagement and corruption continues to be the albatross around their neck, the bureaucratic process complex, and the criteria for support difficult to apply. Nor is there much fiscal space for even well-targeted and administered government support. The way in which much of the funding voted for small businesses ended up in the coffers of big business is an example of just how difficult it is to target such instruments correctly.

Many small businesses did not survive beyond the seven weeks window. Some with strong cash position will rise from the ashes, perhaps even reposition their business to be better attuned to the new landscape. Others will give up and join the job queue. Those with specific skills and knowledge of working in their business may even jump to the front of the new normal return with fresh entrepreneurial activities.

Once the economy returns to growth currently a dim prospect, we do not know the scale of loss suffered by these entrepreneurs. But all would bear the scars of the virus and its terrible twin, the recession. It is ironic that it is not the working of the economy, but rather the shutting down of it that has most starkly exposed our unequal conditions, those at the top of economic ladder own most of everything will flourish while those at the bottom will continue to lick wounds and perhaps perish on their own.

Eighteen million South Africans bring home monthly income average of R2600, which must support on average of five members of the breadwinner's household. In contrast 7 million are in the upper income quintile upwards of R38000 supporting two household members. The ability of these households to withstand the economic effects of a sustained lockdown is like day and night. An economy where 40% of the population share 6% of national income and 39% of people live on a monthly income of R 490 is simply incomprehensible.

There are approximately 5 million workers who earn their livelihood in the informal economy. The closing off the tap that allow them to earn their meagre income has meant being plunged into hunger and even deeper poverty. For most of the migrants, the lockdown meant neither income from informal work nor from COVID-19 grant. With this picture it was not surprising to see the queues for food we have seen in April and May.

'Okay, so you are implying here, what is that?'

'My point is this government can claim anti-racism in its public rhetoric, but it can't claim to be anti-xenophobic in practise. Migrants from Afrikan countries are the only people group excluded from the country's social net.

South Africa's budget deficit stands at 15.7% of GDP and the country is on its way to sovereign debt crisis. This crisis of spiralling public debt is the direct result of years 26 years of crass politics. The debt burden future generations loom large. South Africa's best case is not driving over the cliff of financial ruin but self-preservation.

Consider the case of Christina Mothibi who had always wanted to return home, but not like this. In 2006 she left Laaste Hoop, her village in Limpopo and moved in with her sister in Mondeo, south of Joburg. It took her four years but eventually found a job, as a tea-lady in Malburton shopping centre. In 2015, she was promoted to an administrator. Her salary supported four others: a brother, her mother and two children. There was enough spare cash for a plot in the village. She had hoped to build a house on the land before she retired. Then came the pandemic.

'With this pandemic life is not what it used to be.' says Christina. She was laid off two weeks after the lockdown began. There were no prospects and rent were due, so she left without giving her landlord a notice and went back to her village home. She has shelved her retirement plans and is focused solely on ensuring her family has something to eat. 'You can't understand how stressed I am right now.'

Christina has more prosaic concerns. She worries that there may be no point in trying her luck in Joburg again, even if the pandemic subsides. She is thinking of setting up her fruit and vegetable stand at the local taxi rank to make ends meet. It was not the return to the land she envisaged. 'But I can't sit here and fold my arms.'

Before coronavirus, the country was in its second recession in two years. That dire situation has turned into a disaster. A sense of scale is given by ground-breaking research from an academic consortium, which used data from a mobile phone survey to produce one of the first detailed analyses of the economic effects of the pandemic in this country. The report published in July, show how the pandemic has impoverished South Africa.

According to the research, one in three people who earned an income in February did not earn in April. About half of the erstwhile earners were permanently laid off, rather than furloughed, suggesting that the effects of the pandemic will be long-lasting. South Africa's eye-wateringly high unemployment rate was set to rise even further.

The studies show the uneven effects of the economic restrictions. Researchers reckon that women account for 2 of the 3 million net job losses. Manual labours were nearly three times as likely to have been laid off as professionals. The lockdown also led to mass internal migration. Between end of March and May, five to six million adults left townships and went back to their village homes. Urbanisation has gone into reverse, as people like Christina went back to the villages to reunite with their families. So far, most movers have gone back to cities.

We know that, during the Level 5 lockdown, many such people moved back to their rural homes. If the jobs or informal business opportunities that attracted them to urban areas are gone, how many would give up and rather remain in the relative familiarity of their rural homes rather than starting the search for an urban income afresh?

Rural-urban migration and education often form around sources of income. In rural areas, old age pensions act as a magnet, drawing in the unemployed, the non-economically active and children to what often become granny-headed households, while many other household members are in the cities working or searching for jobs. So, children may remain while parents move to urban areas. The children may later join a parent or parents in the cities, often when entering primary or high school.

While part of the household remains in a rural area, rural pension incomes may be supplemented by child grants and remittances from urban household members. As urban roots grow stronger over time, fewer household members may remain in rural areas. What will happen now that many urban individuals have lost their jobs when they trek back to the rural countryside?

Perhaps this may be true, especially for those who are only a few years below the age of pension-eligibility. On the other hand, remittances may also dry up. And what about the children who have been brought back to the rural areas? It is not clear if all will return to their schools in urban areas. Perhaps we could see some shifts in the school-going population when schools resume, with some rural schools expanding at the expense of urban ones.

But the unemployment rate has been exceptionally high for decades and millions of South Africans have never had a job. Children enter adulthood with the support of a grant and into a labour market of zero opportunities. Jobless returnees have put pressure on families. Of the households that received people in May, most reported that they ran out of money for food. Overall, nearly half of respondents said they could not afford enough food in April more than twice the share of households saying they could not do so at any point during 2017, according to a comparable survey.

The president hopes that the economy will soon recover but there are ample reasons to worry. For starters, the virus surged in July; South Africa was according to the five-day moving averages of case totals collated by John Hopkins University the fifth most affected country in the world at that time. Epidemiological models used by the modelling consortium suggest cases peaked between late August month and end of September, depending on the province.

South Africa was trying to balance surging caseloads with rekindling economic activity. A huge risk. Ramaphosa seems to be siding with the statistics. A tactic he adopted to shore up his position within the party ahead of the ANC's National General Council. But it is because he sees the state as a driver of rather than a brake on growth. At the same time, he echoed the party's other faction, saying that radical economic transformation must underpin the economic future. It is a normal self-serving behaviour of politicians, the need to survive attacks from opponents.

The reform of public health must be speeded up, the government must hasten the phased introduction of the National Health Insurance. There is little needing repair in our economy, its major aspects must be overhaul fundamentally. Starting with the infrastructure the foundations upon which the colonial legacies rests. But in the interim, we need a clear path to recovery so that society can be on its legs ready to work again.

> 'I promise you Brad I will kill anyone I hear saying another word about nine-point this and six-point that. These clowns have been talking about the phantom five-six-seven-point plans for the longest time now, after twenty-six years this is thoroughly boring.

Now, we have invested nothing in re-imagining our economy. At the last count, I think there were several plans to tackle structural unemployment, land reform, a weak schooling and healthcare system for the majority and spatial divides that sentence us to a life lived apart. For more than 26 years, these plans have hit their own roadblocks from either established business and their pained adoption of transformation efforts, or the unions more concerned about monthly subscriptions of the dwindling membership than the welfare of this country. To say nothing of the lying government.

Our greatest advantage is that we've never been satisfied with how we were before the pandemic and for all our political theatre, we've all agreed on the need for change and the plans have been drawn in the pursuit of a just society. Policymakers and corporate titans remain baffled. We need not be, given the work that has already gone into restructuring what country we live in. The winter of discontent will be long great suffering will follow, but in it, I urge that we use this crisis to define who we are with the playbooks we have in the locker room.

Corruption was certainly the antagonist-in-chief over the past decade as it relegated the National Development Plan to a coffee table, an economic blueprint to which we should perhaps cling to at this time. Some are saying we must dust off this plan and rethink solutions because of this presenting crisis.

There are terrible side-effects of the shutdown including the destruction of farming, economic ruin, and poverty. Considering that one of the things that COVID-19 had was affecting some in parts of the country worse than most, exacerbating these with shutdown was counterproductive. There was no point in running from a snake to end up on a cholla cactus. Back up and retreat calmly.

Precious lives and millions of fragile livelihoods have been lost. For many South Africans grimly hanging on and fighting for the survival, news and information alone is not enough. Many who had gambled by embarking on an entrepreneurial career and started new firms or businesses - even successful ones - may not survive the lockdown and the following recession thereafter.'

'But how did you survive the ordeal, your business is hardly four years old?' I asked.
'I regard myself fortunate in that I work in a niche area, that is how I managed to save enough cash to carry the business throughout this time without signing up new contracts.'
'Lucky you.'
'So, the lockdown has affected people differently.'
'Sure.'
'Some have seen their dreams of successful businesses shattered. Many must fall back on that familiar South African last resort, the extended family.'

Now, let me look through a wider lens at the state of the world today. The world economic system is spinning out of control, powerful people are powerless to act to stop the breakdown. Businesses stopped producing goods and services, unemployment rose, people stopped buying goods, stopped travelling, stopped talking, incomes dwindled consequently the world entered a recession possibly deep recession like that experienced in the 1920s. Fear defines their lack of confidence in the world system, and their fear does feed the recessionary mood. With the coronavirus pandemic, the world became vulnerable and fragile.

China will cease to be the global logistics hub many companies have relied upon previously. They will speed up their relocation from China to other developing economies where there is a good infrastructure enabling fast movement of goods. Another factor is that industries that are in decline are low value-added products.

The prevailing attitude is to blame something or somebody. 'It is those people that gave us this disease, let us punish them through economic sanction if this does not work let us attack with our military hardware and smoke them out.' This is a familiar fear-driven refrain during times of crisis. It is said that knowledge is antidote to fear, it is the government's fear rather than facts that dictated how they responded to the pandemic and the subsequent advice they gave to the public.

Those that leaned upon the government have been disappointed. This time things have gone worse. People have become a kakistocracy if you like — a class that is the opposite of aristocrats, those in leadership. South Africa is going to end up a country with permanently lower levels of everything: employment, income, savings, trust, happiness, and assets. Already in the process of becoming a poor country with the failed politics too. Coronavirus has accelerated and finalised the grim transformation into paralysis and total collapse.

Democracy is a luxury. It takes time, money, effort to be a democratic society. A society of servants is rarely a truly democratic one. The ruling class is now visibly made of predators, the kinds of men and women who put men in cages, or addict a whole society to painkillers, just to make more money than they will never spend.

A dying economy is a nation plunging into poverty. A dying economy takes systems and institutions of public good with it. A dying economy takes a functioning society with it, it is norms of trust and acceptance and coexistence and tolerance. And a dying economy, ultimately, takes a sane, decent, sensible politics with it. When an economy dies, everything we cherish and treasure dies. What is really withering is human potential itself.

It may well be that history will judge the president favourably for his people pleasing stance but not for decisiveness. From where I am seating, there is nothing the president did differently that any bus driver could not have done producing the same outcomes without sweating. We expected more from the leadership of this president, fewer deaths, and lessened suffering. We got neither. If you call that success congratulation.

It is a painful irony that the two nations that arguably did the least to prevent COVID-19 deaths, particularly among the most vulnerable, were hailed as the world's two best-prepared before the crisis hit. Clearly, we need to re-examine what preparedness means. Countries that kept their COVID-19 death rates extremely low ranked poorly on the preparedness scorecard issued by a Washington think-tank a year earlier, like

Mongolia (ranked 46), Vietnam (50), and Iceland (58). The catastrophic USA, U.K and RSA responses to the pandemic show that when we give out future grades to countries on how well prepared they are to handle the next pandemic, we need to account for a country's political decision-making as one of the most important determining factors.

There is power in honesty in failure, a down-to-earth confrontation with reality that seem lacking at the highest office in the land. To fully embrace the experience of failure in 2020, not merely to tolerate it as a steppingstone to a better life, is to abandon this childish belief that never to put a foot wrong is possible.

Bro, if there should be areas of disagreement between us, the margin has shrunk appreciably. I can see we have a shared future. I recognise it is late in the day; I suspect you may want to do final touches for your return to work tomorrow. Maybe we can pick up the discussions some other time. Right.' We part ways with a group hug.

'Go well my brother.'

'Travel mercies.' Ayo wishes them.

'Bae, you know what I like about Brad, is his perceptive mind. He can pick up small nuances and turn them into insightful observations. He is incisive with his questions a mark of intelligence. I find him a good challenge. Brad raises his hand and wave goodbye; we wave back at them. The car turns towards the main gate. Sharp halogen lights of the Merc Cabriole shimmer on our faces momentarily turning us into ghost-like figurines. I pull Ayo towards me and thread my right hand into the collar of her windbreaker and let it linger for one, two, three, four… She clings tightly to my arm refusing to release it pinching instead my biceps.

'I love you honey bunch.'

'Dig you lots, Hon.'

Monday, 16th November
Economic recovery, what bollocks?

Zweli Mkhize, the Health Minister appears to have lost a lot of weight since the start of the pandemic considerably so after the touch with COVID-19. It also appears he has become less busy these days because he can be seen taking radio interviews, jogging in the streets, and sparing a moment to join in on #JerusalemaChallenge. During one of radio interviews, he was asked to give an appraisal of the general climate of the lockdown in the land, he described it as 'markedly improved' sounding upbeat seeing bright prospects in the days ahead.

In the follow up explanation in what he thought was a hint to the audience, making a prelude speech foreshadowing what the president was going to announce in shortly thereafter. From the choice of words used he went further than just dropping a hint.

This evening the president is about to take the podium at the Manhlambandlovhu to announce a set of new measures responding to the improving pandemic conditions in the country. As people who have endured the pandemic and resultant lockdown for six months, waiting is one aspect that most of us have been unable to master. To some degree the waiting made us patient, to a greater extent the waiting consumed us. To bide by our time is work for now. It is understandable therefore, that everybody is expecting him to announce something much more hastening relieving us of the boredom.

People want the post-pandemic country that is more sustainable and equitable. A majority wants to see this economy reimagined to be more inclusive. The crisis that disproportionately impacted women followed by a recovery that puts them at the centre. They want to see government, businesses, and organizations including women's voices at all levels of decision-making. And the women whose unsung, underpaid work finally recognized as essential will find new security and opportunity in the world that emerges from the other side.

Today, the president is addressing parliament sharing the government's recovery plan in what is arguably his best attempt responding to the pandemic and its effects on the economy. I manage to catch him when he opened his address, whose extract reads thusly.

> 'What South Africans want from Parliament today is reassurance that we are committed to a swift and inclusive recovery, that we will do whatever it takes and that we have

their best interests at heart. Our challenge is not only to recover to pre-pandemic levels of economic activity, but to lift ourselves out of an economic decline that has been several years in the making, while seeking to undo structural distortions that were many decades in the making. Unlike many other national economies, we have to recover jobs that were lost as we had to shut down much of the economy, but also to alleviate the plight of millions of people who were already jobless before the pandemic hit. To ensure that our efforts are focused, our plan is driven by five key priorities: infrastructure investment and delivery; an employment stimulus; energy security; measures to promote localisation and African integration; and, to improve the capacity of the state. The plan is underpinned by a commitment to fiscal sustainability and economic reforms that will enable growth. It is about choosing a few things and doing them properly. This involves, in the first instance, urgent steps to remove the impediments to investment and greater economic activity. These include fixing our energy challenges, undertaking structural reforms in areas like telecommunications and transport, and improving the ease of doing business. There should be no doubt that this plan aims to unleash the capacity of the private sector to create jobs on a far larger scale and at a greater pace… Through the Presidential Employment Stimulus, we are using a substantial expansion in the scope of public employment programmes to mitigate unemployment and support recovery. Over the next three years, R100 billion in public investment will create hundreds of thousands of work opportunities and support livelihoods in many sectors. We will be boosting existing programmes such as the Expanded Public Works Programme and Community Work Programme. But we will also be innovating on other fronts to create avenues for social employment in communities. Social employment offers income security to those who are of working age but have been unable to find work…. During the past several weeks, we have published an invitation to apply for high-demand spectrum that will enable the modernisation of our telecommunications system. We have made significant progress in our efforts to achieve energy security, activating the process for the procurement of new generating capacity in line with the Integrated Resource Plan and issuing new regulations to allow municipalities in good financial standing to generate their own power. Agreements with Independent Power Producers to expand our generation capacity are being concluded and we are unlocking emergency electricity supply. The 700 000 hectares of state-owned land that we are going to make available to our people is one of the measures that we are embarking upon to fulfil the promise of land redistribution and expand our agricultural production. Making access to land to our people remains one of the key pillars of our developmental and transformative policy approaches to improve the lives of our people… I call on leaders across society to lend your wisdom, your ideas and your encouragement to the National Economic Recovery Council, which will be driving the implementation of this plan.'

The monotonous rumbling went on until I ran out of steam, switched off the damn television. In any case, I am not sure if there is still a single person in this country who believes in dream however hard the government sells it. If there are such people, they know something the rest of us do not, we would appreciate it if they could school us so we could renew our faith again. Accordingly, I will not bother you a word more about the president's dream since I this is a waste of your time and mine.

Tuesday, 1st December
The wonder of vaccines

Waiting for a breakthrough in the fight against COVID-19 has been a bit like waiting for a bus to arrive at remote village of Qaqadu in the mountainous Eastern Cape. In the long dark tunnel that has been 2020, December stands as the month that light appeared. Some say it is a bright light, others see it as a dim light - but unmistakably a light.

Despite the difficulties, science was able to break down barriers between government and industry to produce good news in a year that was otherwise overshadowed by pain and death. Almost a year of waiting, between 31st January 2020 and December, four vaccines came at once, another dozen followed weeks thereafter. That they are all arriving at the same time was a special blessing. The tool the world needed to emerge from the COVID-19 pandemic finally arrived.

Seeing the progress already made, it is outrightly astonishing. Humans have never made more progress on any disease in a year than our present day scientists did on COVID-19. This medical accomplishment is nothing short of a miracle. The estimates of middle 2022 look likely that vaccines will be rolled out globally.

The heroes rose to the occasion and developed effective vaccines with astonishing speed riding on the back of some of the greats. They built on the spectacular discovery by the greats such as Francis Crick, James Watson, Fred Sanger. Molecular genetics is a form of digital information technology on steroids.

Around 15th January, Chinese scientist had typed the genome sequence of the virus. The code for the virus that causes COVID-19 is around 30,000 letters long. Compared to influenza viruses, which are made up of eight genetic segments that can be rearranged in lots of different ways the coronavirus is a much simpler virus. The most notable mutations we've seen so far have happened in the same spot, the spike protein on the surface of the virus.

That limited capacity for change may explain why we keep seeing the same mutations appear in different places rather than lots of distinct variations. Both B.1.1.7 first detected in the UK and B.1.351 first detected in South Africa evolved independently, yet they share a number of the same mutations. The key will be genetic sequencing in combination with better disease surveillance. If we don't get the vaccine out to every corner of the planet, we'll have to live with the possibility that a much worse strain of the virus is likely to emerge soon. It is possible to see a new variant emerge that evades the first generation vaccines altogether.

It took BioNTech 3 days to computer-model their vaccine. It took Moderna 63 days to design and formulate their mRNA. From to the lab desktop to late-stage human trials, the world was given its first vaccine in ten months flat. It was rushed. This we recognised, in doing so scientist missed (in some instances were told) to eliminate crucial aspects of the design and trial phase in the race to defeat the virus.

By beginning of November Pfizer/BioNTech announced that they had developed a safe and effective vaccine for the illness. A week later Moderna announced that it too has developed a vaccine that is equally safe and effective. The following week was the turn of Gamaleya to put a spotlight on its Sputnik V vaccine telling the world it has achieved the same efficacy standards as the rival American vaccine producers.

Sinopharm the Chinese producer never bothered with the stupid PR stunt, they simply went ahead with the clinical trials and when they got the statistically important 95% confidence level they needed, were granted the emergency approval by the Chinese government and started the immunization programme of one million of its soldiers. Then after clinical trials in other settings told the world about their results.

The road was smoothed for all the necessary paperwork ahead of time, and they were already drawing up plans for the logistics when the vaccine would be finally distributed to the countries that bought it early.

The second wave infections threatened to dither economies for the second time, this accelerated the pace of clinical trials. Aided by a confluence of three factors. A new technology of developing vaccines was already in the pipeline waiting to be tested following the MERS outbreak, with the coronavirus becoming the perfect target.

How vaccines work

Vaccine work by attacking the same part of the protein that has its crown-like shape. Because the spike protein is what attaches to human cells, thus allowing the virus to enter. Researchers know that attacking this protein work. Scientists have had this in mind when they formulated the vaccines. The vaccines train our immune systems to recognise the spike protein.

By blocking this entrance infection is prevented. The immune system develops antibodies that block the spike protein of the virus's surface, and the infected person is protected from severe COVID-19. These vaccines do nothing to produce the longer staying T-cells soldiers of the body.

A vaccine does not give hundred percent cure but offers effective protection from severe COVID-19 illness. In fact, vaccines do not protect against infection neither do they prevent transmission. They block symptoms from appearing. As a result, vaccinated people can carry and spread pathogens without knowing it. Occasionally, they can even start new epidemics when they have mutated into a new strain.

Types of immunity

There are two main types of immunity that can be achieved with vaccines. Effective immunity acts to prevent a pathogen from causing serious illness but cannot stop it from entering the body. Then there is sterilising immunity, this type can stop infections entirely, and even prevent asymptomatic cases. The 2nd generation vaccines, it is hoped, would deliver the promise of sterilizing immunity. The world must keep an eye on this technology. I am a keen student.

To achieve sterilising immunity, the second generation vaccines must stimulate enough of the antibodies to catch any virus particles entering the body and immediately disarm them.

Panicked by the impact this would have on their countries' economy, governments of the world were willing to do more whatever it took to deliver the vaccine before its maturity time. So far, the available vaccines have not been designed primarily to prevent transmission instead, they are made to prevent mild to moderate symptoms from developing into severe disease. This means that the drug makers set their targets low because of the feared economic damage.

Scientists already knew by the end of 2020 that antibodies people develop after infections with COVID-19 don't always prevent them from being reinfected. One study of British healthcare workers found that 17% of those who had antibodies already when the study began – presumably from a first infection – caught it a second time. Around 66% of these cases were asymptomatic.

They eliminated financial risks for the pharma companies and streamlined administrative roadblocks standing in the way of approvals and even allowing production to begin before late-stage trials were completed with the critical final data evaluated in-situ. Literally, they threw money at this challenge. Beside governments like China, US and Germany, the group called the Coalition for Epidemic Preparedness Innovation, funded by Melinda & Gates foundation and several other philanthropic foundations helped to speed up things.

Governments run countries as though they were corporations driven by a profit motive. Shutting down the economy for the second time was a risk none were prepared to take because that would have meant their ratings would plummet and the prospects of their re-elections goes down with it. Governments announced vaccines while still in the lab several months before the thing was even ready to go phase III clinical trials the late-stage human testing, that is how desperate the times were. Everybody wanted to get the solution for this thing however it was defined.

Seven 1st generation vaccine candidates had emerged as front runners undergoing early approval in various jurisdictions including China, Russia, USA,

Germany, France, and UK. The companies responsible for designing and manufacturing these vaccines are BioNTech/Pfizer (BNT162b2, 95% effective), Moderna (mRNA1273, 94,5% effective, Oxford University/AstraZeneca (AZD1222, 70.4% effective), Gamaleya (Sputnik V, 91.4%), Novavax (NVX-CoV2373), Sinopharm (Coronavac, 81% effective) Johnson & Johnson (ENSEMBLE, 81%) and Sinovac Biotech (CoronaVac). Late comers of the 1st generation included CanSino Biologics (Ad5nConV) and Sanofi/GSK(MRT5500).

An ideal vaccine is one that is safe with mild, transient side effects e.g. low-grade fever. It should confer long-lasting protection of more than one season to more than 80% of the population. It should protect not only against disease but prevent virus transmission to others as well. And ideally, it should be administered as a single dose.

It should be able to be produced quickly and in large quantities. It should be easily stored not at ridiculously ultra-low temperatures. It should be easily transported outside of the cold-chain or even through the mail and it should be easily administered without requiring special devices or administered by those without training.

It is important to note we are unlikely to have a vaccine that is perfect offering all the advantages expected of a vaccine. It is good enough if a vaccine can satisfy the safety shortly after vaccination and in the long term protect a substantial proportion of those vaccinated against severe disease, particularly those in the most vulnerable groups with underlying medical conditions. Assuming that 70 percent of the world's population must be immunised to break transmission, the world will have to manufacture 10 billion of two-dose vaccines. Here are some of the first past-the-post vaccines approved in December 2020.

Types of vaccines

Sinopharm/Wuhan Biological Products Research Institute and Sinovac Biotech's vaccines uses the inactivated method where the virus is inactivated so that it can no longer replicate. The inactivated virus stimulates the body's immune system to produce antibodies so when a person is exposed to the actual virus, antibodies are called to action to fight the virus.

This method is well-established in the production of vaccines. Inactivated virus vaccines include vaccines against influenza, polio, hepatitis A, and rabies viruses. Viral vaccines require booster doses to achieve a sustain protection. Although inactivated vaccines typically do not provide immune responses as strong as attenuated or weakened viruses, they do prevent moderate to severe illness from viral infections.

Protein-based vaccines

Sanofi/GSK and SpyBiotech partnership are producing vaccines introducing proteins from the virus itself including viral proteins whole or just pieces of it but without genetic material and then together with an adjuvant trigger an immune response with lasting immunity. The Novavax vaccine for example, uses nanoparticles from the soap bark tree to deliver viral proteins to cells of the immune system and stimulate strong immune responses. Protein-based vaccines are combined with additives in small quantities that improve immune responses. These protein-based vaccines work much like inactivated vaccines by exposing the immune system to viral proteins and inducing protective immune responses without causing the disease in humans.

Protein-based vaccines include vaccines for hepatitis B virus, shingles, and the bacteria that causes whooping cough. Vaccines with adjuvants cause local reactions such as redness, swelling, and pain at the injection site, and more systemic reactions such as fever, chills, and body aches than non-adjuvanted vaccines.

Vector vaccines

Oxford University/AstraZeneca, Johnson & Johnson and Gamaleya use non-replicating virus that deliver genes in the into human cells where viral proteins are produced to induce protective immune responses. However, the Sputnik V vaccine uses both human and chimpanzee adenoviruses as vectors. The weakened vectors do not replicate because important genes have been deleted. The viral DNA is not integrated into the host genome but is copied into messenger RNA and translated into proteins. The vaccine uses a chimpanzee adenovirus as vector, thus minimizing the risk of pre-existing immunity to the vector that might reduce vaccine efficacy.

Viral vectors have been studied for several decades for gene therapy, to treat cancer, and for research into molecular biology. Viral vectors other than adenoviruses include retroviruses and the vaccinia virus that was used to prevent smallpox. In July 2020, the European Commission approved use of an adenovirus 26 vaccine for Ebola the first adenovirus vectored vaccine approved for use in humans. Adenoviruses are a group of common viruses that can cause cold-like symptoms, fever, sore throat, diarrhoea, and pink eye. These vaccines require two doses.

Genetic vaccines

Moderna/NIAID, BioNTech/Pfizer, CureVac/ICL uses the latest technology of mRNA vaccines. The mRNA approach is regarded as particularly important scientific breakthrough because this is the first successful example of a new class of drugs that work by feeding cells message to turn the body's cell into vaccine-making bodies. Gene therapy acts as the software programming to the body's immune system hardware and primes immune cells to recognize and attack the viral genetic material.

The RNA does not need to get into the nucleus. It simply needs to be delivered into the more accessible outer region of cells, the cytoplasm, which is where proteins are constructed. This vaccine delivers the spike protein gene directly into the human cells as RNA instead of using a vector to deliver genes to human cells. mRNA vaccines are taken up into cells, but do not enter the nucleus, which then induce immune responses. The vaccines encapsulate the mRNA in tiny oily capsules, known as lipid nanoparticles. Nanoparticles are more stable and do not have to be stored at extremely low temperatures.

DNA contains the codes for all of the proteins our bodies are made up of. The recipes contained in DNA are translated via an intermediary called messenger-RNA. mRNA then joins with another cell component called a ribosome that uses the code in the mRNA to construct the desired protein by collecting and combining amino acids into the finished product.

mRNA vaccines are not going to affect your DNA. Cells' genome is contained within the nucleus of the cell, which is surrounded by a double-membrane. It allows for molecules such as mRNA to leave but blocks molecules from entering it. So, the S-protein mRNA from the vaccine will not enter the nucleus until it is broken down into nucleotides. Even if the mRNA molecule could affect the DNA, there are all kinds of error correction machinery in the DNA to keep out random bits of code.

With trillions of cells in each human, each containing billions of DNA base pairs, the DNA keep close watch over errors. The mRNA from the mRNA vaccines do not interact with the DNA in any way. They cause the ribosome to produce the S-protein antigen, and that's it. Once a copy of the molecule of S-protein is produced at the ribosome from one strand from the vaccine, that mRNA strand is broken down into individual nucleotides to be reused by the cell.

The exploitation of messenger RNA to produce coronavirus spike proteins to which the body responds by making neutralizing antibodies is a clever way of inducing an immune response without the need for a preceding infection. In addition, mRNA could in future be used, as BioNTech and Moderna are pioneering, to fight cancer. Harnessing a process called immunotherapy, the mRNA can be coded to produce molecules that will cause the body's immune system to identify and kill cancer cells. In 2018, a young Chinese doctor used CRISPR to engineer twin girls, so they did not have the receptor for the virus that causes AIDS. There was an immediate awe and then expressions of ethical concerns. Officials denounced the young scientist. But in the wake of the pandemic, RNA-guided genetic editing to make humans less receptive to viruses will soon be more acceptable as mainstream. That day may be tomorrow. Watch the space.

The success of the mRNA vaccines bodes well for dealing with any future mutations of sars-cov-2. The different vaccine types are not interchangeable. Once a country selects a vaccine, the same vaccine is used for a second dose. There will not be enough to protect everyone at first yet getting the shots to the right people could change the course of the pandemic. Vaccine supplies will be limited to frontline workers, then health care workers in essential industries, then people with pre-existing medical conditions and grannies over the age 60.

The impact

The coronavirus won't ever be stamped out, it will become one of the many seasonal viruses that infects people. In the meantime, if you are immunized, you can still get infected with the virus and pass it on to others but less likely to get sick. If everyone were vaccinated with 95% effective vaccines today, theoretically COVID-19 would cease to be a public health emergency within months following the introduction of a vaccine. In reality a different picture emerged. The pandemic would be expected to end having achieved true herd immunity around 80% of the population. A mutation that makes humans less ill will spread faster but not more deadly. This virus will evolve and eventually give us no more than a cold, like several other coronaviruses have already done in the past.

The wait is not over

Even with the best science available, there are many unknown variables we must deal with; no one knows when this pandemic is going to end or how. COVID-19 is a new disease, and there is no way for predicting its future. No one knows how long it will take the world to reach herd immunity or whether we will get there at all since the virus mutates faster than vaccines can be administered. Scientists do not know how many people need to get vaccinated to reach the required threshold. Even if everything goes well, there will always be people who choose not to be vaccinated. Plus, children younger than 16 are currently not eligible for vaccination. This is a daunting goal.

The president told us in November that we were due to get a vaccine and has set aside R300 million from the Solidarity Fund. In December he updated the nation saying 'I only know of R250 million available to pay for vaccines. We are busy evaluating many vaccines at the moment, we are likely to get ours sometime in February 2021.' February moved to April then to May. This is when our winter season starts, even then it will be enough for the frontline health workers. We know the president is counting himself and his friends and their families to receive this jab reserved for the frontline people. You and I will be lucky if we get vaccinated at all. We may have to buy our own in the end.

The world has received and distributed the COVID-19 vaccines to their citizens but not so for South Africa. The government, in addition, to making late payment mistakenly relying on the goodwill and benevolence of high-income countries to share the Covax network an act that exposed South Africa's ineptitude. Government has reinforced my observation of not being in the game they are unable to escape their own incompetence the best they could do was to save their skin. Anyone believing otherwise must be crazy.

South Africa promised to vaccinate 1.25 frontline health workers within a short space of time but faltered taking longer to do so. Government announced phase two starting middle of May without completing phase one of the programme. Even after vaccines are available for mass immunization, Epidemiologists estimate that it could take six months to achieve the 67% inoculation required to achieve herd immunity in best run health systems like the UK. South Africa could take much longer than a year to achieve the same status. Best case scenario is that we would be 'safe' from June 2022.

The first shipment of the vaccine mark just the beginning of what is a long and messy road. It is going to be a slow process especially that the government is considering the use of an online self-enrolment portal called electronic vaccine data system for pre-booking and issuance of vaccine certificates. The biggest confusion is bound to be around the two vaccine distribution systems one for Medical Aids (the insured) administered by private GPs and Dis-Chem.

A different distribution for the uninsured folks via community clinics. But the government says it will contract Dis-Chem and other large-scale pharmacies including GPs to provide a vaccine for the uninsured. The hard work begins now because not everybody is settled on the idea of a vaccine. Safe or not. Only 60% of South Africans have shown the desire to take a vaccine. The question must be asked what would happen to those who cannot produce a vaccination card on demand when they find new employment or must travel abroad?

Everything depends on whether the world comes together to ensure that the lifesaving science developed in 2020 saves as many lives as possible in 2021 and beyond. Until vaccines reach everyone in the world new clusters of disease will continue popping up. For this reason, the guideline remains that for 2021 and beyond people must continue to wear a mask in public, practice social distancing and avoid large indoor gatherings until this thing has blown over not just in South African but the world over, then the pandemic will be over, remaining instead with endemic presence of COVID-19.

Thursday, 7th January
Everybody said it was going to be a 'new normal'

There have been worse years in South African history, and certainly worse years in world history, but most of us alive today have seen nothing like this one. Our most debilitating threat this year was a sense of helplessness, and it ran unchecked. Helplessness met its evil twin, a partner that would only magnify its mad power: isolation. So many didn't have that privilege and lost their jobs, with no means to pay their rent and no way to feed their families. Hunger became a major theme of 2020, presenting challenges even in countries with the means to assuage it.

At the same time, parents no matter their means, hustled to take care of and home school their kids. Meanwhile, front-line workers, from grocery store helpers to truck drivers to hospital nurses and doctors, continued to show up for duty. I have seen clips of health care workers in the news, their faces marked by hours of wearing PPE, their eyes leaden with weariness.

Sometimes unable to hold back tears, they'd describe a new addition to their daily routine: watching patients die when they could no longer keep them alive. At a designated time, each evening some in other parts of the world leaned out of their windows, armed with pots and wooden spoons or just our oddball cacophony of human voices, and raised a ruckus in solidarity with front-line workers. It was the least we could do, at a time when we had no idea what else to do.

That began in March, the onset of a period in which most of us felt encased in our own lonely bubbles, looking out at a world that seemed to be falling apart. We played board games and did jigsaw puzzles and really talked and listened to our children. All of those are undoubtedly good things, and we nod in solemn agreement when our neighbours enumerate those blessings.

But none of them capture the micro-texture of what our lives were like this year. In the cities, when we were told we should not go out at all except for occasional exercise, walks in the sunshine became the thing we hung onto. How lucky we were to be able to do that, at least!

In the suburbs, our restricted routines opened new routes of creativity: we might drive out of our way to catch a spectacular sunset, or finally tackle a hiking trail we'd always meant to explore. Then came the time when it became possible to meet a friend for a takeout glass of wine.

This became the summer of lukewarm and acidic rosé in a plastic cup, but it represented a privilege and a pleasure that, in earlier months, we weren't sure we'd have. For that reason, perhaps many of us have felt through 2020 that it's easier to connect with old art than with new.

The bromides are already flowing freely. We slowed down. All manner of amusements has been streamed right into our homes, some of them quite wonderful. Because nearly all of our movie blockbusters and big year-end spectacles were cancelled, we spent more time watching stories about human beings talking to one another rather than chasing down a bunch of magic stones from a bejewelled glove.

Even so, very little of what we watched helped us make sense of this moment. We were bored, anxious or, worse, unemployed. We've had lots of time to get to know ourselves better, which often leaves us more bewildered and less trusting of our judgment. We were drained. We give up and watch The Office again, though there are worse things.

This was not the time to be hard on ourselves for not knowing exactly what we want, except to continue to remain hidden from the virus to stay alive, and to do what we can to make sure the same goes for our neighbours and loved ones. We were tired with good reason. This virus attacks the weakest and most vulnerable and has thus disproportionately affected certain portions of the population.

All the rules and restrictions have made us weary, yet it was more important than ever to be vigilant. For now, members of our families, friends whom we love dearly, people we've never met but whose work has touched us continue to die. The virus is a blanket problem that hits all of us in painfully personal, targeted ways. Will it hold? It will be morning in another day, in the meantime, we have to get through the darkest hour just before. The aurora bides its time.

We learned a lot in 2020 but what, exactly, did we learn? The question where to from here presupposes educated choices on our part. So, when we remind ourselves and each other that we will get back to normal, which normal are we talking about or we must choose from? Is there even such a thing as a new normal, better normal or escape the norm?' 'What are your thoughts.'

'Coronavirus has changed the meaning of many things. It has ruptured a sense of easy normality, placidity, and stability. That things could just go on ad infinitum. Now we know how quickly life can come to a screeching halt with a knock-on effect on everything else. But there can be no mistaking the crucial lesson of this pandemic.

Coronavirus will probably define this decade sapping the life from economies, causing a depression here, a stagnation here, something over there and draining the cohesion from societies overall. As people grow tired of yet another lockdown, shifting power to authoritarians. Corona caused our lives to come to a standstill in more ways than one.

I am not sure, I heard lot of folks talk glibly about this concept. What I do know is this, when people are bored, they are inventive. It may well be another social construction we invented during our moment of inactivity. I have heard many define normal either in statistical, aspirational or functional terms. There is one small problem though, there is a better normal for the elite and privileged like me and there is a bad normal for the rest, the excluded and marginalised like you.

The new normal for the privileged people is qualitatively better. It means that most us will go back to most of what we were doing before the pandemic struck. Kind of wanting to go back to where we were, but also kind of do not. We want things to be the same, but we also want them to be better. We want to return to *our* normal. Perhaps, our journey will not be a return so much as a departure.

Presented with this kind of fluidity therefore, the definition of normal might not be precise, therein lies my difficult to explicate. I am certain though its function is clear: normal is safe. It is the familiar.

We do not begin with normality and then categorise those instances where it is transgressed. We begin with all those things that we instinctively feel are 'abnormal' then try to find comfort by erecting a norm that resolves our anxieties around them. We then locate this norm in this past, which gives us the benefit of claiming the norm as our own. It is not something we want to build from scratch; all that is necessary is that we return home to it.

Most of us thought that once lockdown ended, we'd return to normal, albeit wearing masks, which for many people are inconvenient. The community will never make changes for the better, whatever we end up doing it might just be the preservation of what we have. There will be a return to what we know.

Habits that were part of our previous normality, situations in which it is very difficult to maintain the necessary precautions to avoid an infection, and which reflect the real problem: we still think that the pandemic is just passing through. We're not facing a second wave: we're still in the first, and the way we do most things remains unchanged. Ignoring the advice of scientists for holding back the return to normal is simply creating the conditions for a sustained crisis.

I am nostalgic. Nostalgia for me is originally a longing for a different place after COVID-19 but as time progressed this hankering for something became a longing for a different time, more specifically, for a time that never was. All we have these days is time. Plenty of it can take our minds to nostalgic places. That too, we have in abundance. Nostalgia about eating out, free from anxiety over whether that extra helping of golden fries comes with coronavirus. Perhaps a yearning to get back to the gym. Soft memories of our children before they transformed into feral woodland creatures under the lockdown.

Ultimately, as I came to realise nostalgia was a romance with my own fantasy. Maybe it is that I feel more entitled to stability, comfort, convenience, and pleasure than I ought to. Now, more than ever, I want to cling to nostalgia. For many it may be the only lifebuoy we have in these dark times, as we drift further away from previous life. If we never return to that old normal, my disappointment at being robbed of a chance to experience live music is undiminished.

Perhaps if there is something to hold onto in all of this, it is not my definition of normality but my insistence on saying we will. I am not sure what exactly the future will look like. That we will always be the norm not only of humanity, but of all life. In one sense, there cannot be a return to normal. Our years of navel gazing may in the end prove nothing useful than I thought.

This pandemic goes far beyond masks, hydro-alcoholic gels or lockdowns. The change we need will not come overnight. But the sooner we understand it, the sooner we can demand that politicians design and implement it, the sooner we can start dealing with it, and the sooner we may realise that, though we don't yet believe it, the world has changed, before our eyes, in a few months. And when your world changes, if you insist on continuing to do things as before, it is not going to end well.

Henri Bergson the French philosopher pondered this question when he used the term *elan vital* to describe the mysterious impulse towards an open future that seems to animate all life. Bergson says, 'since its inception, life has been the continuation of one and the same impetus which separates itself into diverging lines of evolution.' Whatever it is, however, we name it, it seems to always be 'we will.'

※ ※

Given that the virus won't change its habits, and that any vaccine we are able to get with won't be a hundred percent cure, the only alternative is to change our ways of thinking. Change our way of life. Start thinking in ways we did not before March 2020. A new redesign, often radical, of many of our activities.

The pandemic requires us to redesign the economy, rethink our obsession with growth, find ways to protect the most vulnerable, use apps to trace our contacts, share research and learning, and redesign everything to put people, not profits first. Cities, restaurants, public spaces, travel, prisons, supply chains, health care, trade, education, work, communication an enormous change that, obviously, the vast majority of the population has yet to imagine.

The only alternative we have and I'm talking the only alternative, not a menu to choose from, is to redesign our lives based on a new reality that will be with us for many years. Until we understand that, we will continue to alternate phases of containment with phases of expansion, all the while waiting for a recovery that in all likelihood will continue to be a mirage, and in the meantime, we'll continue dying like bed bugs. Either we change our mentality and get a grip now or we must die in our foolishness.

Our new normal will be different, though, not because of the social consequences of it. Some things will never be done like before because we will have discovered different and often better ways to do them. An example is the reliance on the digital platforms such on-line shopping that has taken off like crazy. Many people who didn't do on-line shopping before, have been pushed to try it and liked it so much that they are likely use it more often in the future.

What we know about this coronavirus pandemic is that it will fundamentally change how we conduct business domestically and across the globe. The lockdown provided us with an opportunity to press a pause-and-reset button for something new or at least different than what we have been doing before as business community. This pause has created space to think things in anew. With this comes human meditation. South Africa has a rare opportunity to seize the moment. Fresh economic opportunities beckon in coronavirus crisis.

Getting the economy back on its feet calls for investment in whole new climate-friendly infrastructures that boosts growth and creates different jobs as well as different consumption patterns. A unique chance to steer the economy away from carbon economy at much lower financial, social, and political cost has presented itself. Are we ready to take it this opportunity?

The energy sector more broadly and electricity sector specifically stands in a transition space between old and new. South Africa has effectively entered an era that can best be described as electric economy; in which soon there will be no coal and no petrol or gas used in the generation of power for moving equipment and goods. The renewable energy buzz is in vogue. This presupposes the emergent forms of energy that are carbon neutral, self-renewing, and are available in a sustainable way, there is truth in the assumption but the assumption itself is meaningless if cannot be acted upon.

We have a long history of coal-led development, built on extractive mining operations, embedded in the country's painful, racist labour laws, and unequal resource allocation. As things stand, Eskom still enjoys virtual monopolistic power, has a history that is inextricable from apartheid's lack of transparency that has long shielded it from public accountability.

Eskom should not fail, yet Eskom has failed, and South Africa cannot afford and have begun to pay a heavy price for this failure. South Africa's electricity crisis requires broad participation of people and not dominance of politicians and funders.

As we have moved into the nth period of rolling blackouts since 2008, we are all aware of the effects of the lights going off, on households, neighbourhood safety, businesses, economic productivity and life in general. If we are to overcome our climate change challenges means we must grab this opportunity with both hands. Organisations in the different space of the value chain are critical to Eskom's on-going survival.

There is an urgent need to access accurate information, surface critical questions, and facilitating spaces for engagement between stakeholders in the energy sector. We especially need to explore policy evolution and bottom-up innovation for a sustainable energy transition. The renewed interest in CO_2 neutral and climate-friendly energy sources has engendered demand for renewable technologies and a path towards a cleaner world is now within sight, a development that must be welcomed.

Sipho Kings, an environmental writer on sustainability has predicted what would South Africa look like in 21 years from today if it continued its carbon emission path and explains why it would be hell. On the current path, Gauteng emerged during the gold rush in the last century will soon become a desert, a mine dump with no drinkable water, no food security, failing grid infrastructure, poverty-stricken city dwellers will become viciously lawless.

In any case, things have been on a downward trajectory in this country for many years now. Unless the country does something now, something it has never done before, life as we know it today will be forever changed. By 2040 South Africa is going to be destroyed not by bad policies but by self-serving choices preceded by cataclysmic decisions.

The world had started falling apart long before: horrific Australian bushfires had been raging for months and would not be quelled until midyear–just in time for wildfire season in the American West, with its own brazen cycle of devastation. Pictures from either of these scenes–unsettling orange skies in normally paradisiacal parts of California, aerial views of doomy plumes of smoke covering the Australian landscape– would feel apocalyptic in any year.

But in 2020, with so many of us hunkered down inside, it was particularly alarming to reckon with the fragility of the natural world. To think of it burning away not least because we humans have failed it with our poor stewardship invites despair.

Even so, our secondary systems still work by and large. That's not to say we have great systems or even good ones but mostly, they were kept functioning by luck. By systems I refer to the social and financial systems - from healthcare to pensions to banks. These are secondary systems that depend on the deeper primary systems. Next time what is going to be different is that the secondary systems will simply stop functioning.

Let me take a stab at a future in which the progression of rot is allowed to fester. A decade from now, by the 2030s, climate change is going to worsen. From relatively mild to catastrophic. And as it does, where it does, when it does, so too, all those systems we depend on will simply rupture and break. Suddenly. Just like coronavirus did in 2020. The difference tomorrow will be that the secondary systems will come halt, not just our access to them. They will be offline, broken, paralyzed and of no use to the nation.

What happens when a country burn? But by the 2030s, though, we won't be so lucky. Megafires will be a regular unstoppable event raging through hills and plains.

Who's going to pay for the costs of repairing burned homes, schools, offices, clinics? Nobody.

Just like we have rust belt towns today places that are left bare by deindustrialization so too we'll have fire belt towns and villages tomorrow. Just like rust belt towns have been abandoned, so tomorrow's fire belt will be uninhabitable. And the exodus fleeing from it will break whatever is left of the secondary systems. Of course, some places will be lucky, and they'll escape much of this damage.

The losers will be immense in number, and our systems simply don't have the capacity to provide, to offer them income, shelter, housing, medicine, food. What happens then? Welcome to the Climate Depression of the 2030s. It will be much worse than the Great Depression of the 1930s. Since huge chunks of the country are now the fire belt, portions of humanity have nowhere to live, nothing to subsist on, and no way to earn a living. Demand falls and the vicious cycle of falling incomes and lower employment sets in with a vengeance.

Life in Gauteng will by the 2040s begin to keel over from the bottom. Its great towers and chains of life will crash and topple, having had the roots and foundations ripped out. All the little things will be dying off fastest and first insects, bees, fish, and worms which all the chain and ladders of subsistence depend on them.

Who's going to turn the soil when the worms are gone? Who's going to clean the rivers from turning to mud, when the fish are gone? Who's going to nourish the plants that keep the forests healthy when the insects are gone? Now the primary systems the most fundamental one begin to break end up crashing.

Those systems now begin to break down. The soil turns to dust and no harvest or food. Now you have to compete just for food. The rivers turn to mud because the fish are gone. Now clean water becomes a luxury. Raw materials become inaccessible. What happens then? The price of all these things simply skyrocket. And having supply of them will seem like a luxury. Now the collapse of our civilization's primary systems of energy, air, food, water, and medicine becomes inevitable. Energy, air, food, water, medicine the things which keep us clean, nourished, fed, watered, alive in the most basic way.

Is there anyone who knows how to engineer an ocean back together and the rain forest? Neither do I. Once they are gone, we are toast. As those critical resources begin to deplete our systems must crash. How do you price food or water when there's nothing from the around? Nobody cares now even if you have money, because money is just the polite fiction of a civilized society.

Now all that matters is power, and the will to use it. Now things break down in a big way. Nations fall apart and towns turn on one another. The idea of democracy comes to an end, and tribalism, factionalism, every kind of superstition replaces it. All that works is everyone against everyone else and each tribe for themselves. A desperate battle for the life-giving stuff left ensues.

Coronavirus pandemic, in its own way, is preparing us for that. It is trying to teach us how not to end as a civilization. By taking care of one another. Invest now in the things we will need tomorrow. Water, energy, air, food and medicine. Where do they come from? From the earth, the forests, skies and the oceans. Do it now. Do it like never before. People must lay aside their petty squabbles and pointless pursuits. By putting down the remote control, the phone, the drug, the fix and start thinking about how they are going to save the earth so that the earth can continue to provide for them.

Corona is a warning from the end of human civilization, backwards in time. It teaches us how people can see the end from here. They can see the lights going out. The lights of civilization, democracy, freedom, justice, truth, beauty, goodness. All incinerated by the fire, drowned by the flood, and all that is left is a desperate, struggle through the mud and ashes by a very weakened nation. It sucks to live at the end of human civilization. Not just because life is intense then but because you know you can do something to save the earth today. Maybe this is life's only way to teach you that first you must burn so you will know that heat is no child's play. You get it.

Despite this fact the government has no sense of strategic direction or the capacity to re-imagine a better future for this nation. Our individual capability to re-imagine the shared futured cannot be mortgaged to the next generation however lofty our promises sound.'

※ ※

'You know what else I learned while I was down in Platt. There is an emergent shift on the horizon. The gig economy is disappearing giving way to hustle economy. I am not just talking the survivalist hustlers, way down in the food chain the LSM 2 mass market. No Bro, this thing is taking off big in the burbs.'

Unemployed teachers, cooks, dancers are turning to Patreon, Twitch, and we have nothing to sell besides physical touch. The thought jarred me awake all night. Briggle had owned a massage studio, it kept her from eating in the first week of the shutdown when she lost six kilos fretting over the sudden collapse of her business, she'd built up her entire adult life.

She grew the operation from a pop-up in her house to a mini empire with a wall of local best of awards. But when the president closed businesses in March 26, Briggle realised in an instant it could all be over. Her bills were more than R5,000 per month, and it wasn't as if she could give massages from home. 'I had nothing, literally nothing, Briggle said. And this is my life's work. I spent the entire first week crying. What else could I do about it?'

Then, in the second week of the shutdown, during a consultation with a local business advisor, she was asked if she'd ever considered a Patreon. As the consultant explained, the digital-subscription platform once home mainly to YouTubers and

Podcast hosts had also become an ad hoc safety net for thousands of teachers, cashiers, line cooks, and hairstylists who lost work with the onset of stay-at-home orders.

And so Briggle, a mother of two with no previous aspirations to 'influence' online, swiped on some mascara and filmed a three-minute stretching video over the off-screen clatter of someone washing dishes. Access to that video, and the 40 others she has since posted to Patreon, requires a monthly subscription of either R50 or R100. More than 50 people have bought those subscriptions, netting Briggle a monthly pay out. It's not enough, but Briggle says it helps.

The Coronavirus pandemic crushed vast swaths of the economy, slashing consumer demand, closing businesses, and vaporizing millions of jobs. But it's been good to the nascent sliver of the digital economy that helps people channel their existing skills into sellable services. Such services range from eBooks and meal plan templates to online classes, podcasts, membership clubs, newsletters, and porn. They proliferate on platforms including Patreon, Twitch, Substack, Etsy, Teachable, Knowable, Podia, Thinkific, Supercast, Lulu, Outschool, OnlyFans, and Gumtree.

These platforms generally take a cut of each sale made, ranging from 5% to 50%, or charge a recurring fee to sellers for accessing their market. Tech investors have dubbed this the passion economy, a place where anyone can profit doing what she loves. But because that term risks both exaggerating the payoffs of this work and obscuring its ties to the gig economy, the last great labour disruption, we might better call it the hustle economy. An online labour market in which platform-dependent workers create and monetize their own digital products.

Workers in the hustle economy need a platform to succeed. But their work is individualized, self-directed, and on their own schedule. One creator can't substitute for another. The hustle economy is also not new. Tech investors have dubbed this the passion economy, a place where anyone can profit doing what she loves. And since then a wave of new start-ups has launched to capitalize on this model of internet-powered entrepreneurship.

Hustle economy platforms represent an opportunity to commoditize a once-worthless or near-worthless resource. Every person on earth has some deep knowledge or experience or skill in something, she argues. If platforms can funnel that into a product that consumers want, then the value of the hustle economy balloons into the hundreds of millions.

For workers, the premise of hustle economy work is equally seductive. Just like gig work, you can choose your own hours. But with the hustle economy, you can really be your own boss, and spend time only on projects you like and feel proud of. While both the gig economy and conventional employment stripped workers of their autonomy and agency, hustle economy platforms empower them.

Better yet, amid a protracted economic crisis, hustle economy work offers a safety net a second income independent of a corporate employer, or even the physical environment. If Patreon and its ilk once promised flexibility or the chance to do what you love, they now also promise workers like Briggle an income the next crisis can't interrupt.

People see how fragile their connection to the economy is. Their job could go at any second. In the past three months, the baseline for this industry accelerated by 10 years. Workers often flock to alternative work during economic downturns. But if the pandemic also acclimates consumers to new digital products and new relationships with the workers who make them then the shift could prove more permanent.

This time could be different, it's a temporary crisis, at least until we have herd immunity or a vaccine, but the way people do business is going to change. We're already seeing that. Patreon the inarguable granddaddy of hustle economy platforms, founded in 2013 fewer than 140,000 people made any money before the pandemic, according to the analytics site Graphtreon.

That was the case for James Fraser and Jessica Overton, professional ballet dancers from South Africa who now live in Australia. The couple launched a YouTube channel in 2016, where for several years they posted travel vlogs and performance videos. But the channel never quite broke through, and they gradually stopped uploading new material. The pandemic prompted them to try again, but with a discrete product: online ballet classes for aspiring professional dancers.

The two film them on their days off from The Australian Ballet, where they have worked since January, and post the classes to Patreon. We just didn't have any rush or incentive. Coronavirus kind of forced us to start… We wanted a safety net. In Knysna, Kerry Crowley, a 25-year-old sports reporter, launched a long-planned Teachable class about journalism after his company announced furloughs. He has made more than R4,000 for roughly 200 hours of work.

Across the country, 18-year-old Kenzie, an aspiring teacher, left her job at Lowe's to teach on Outschool, a live course platform for grade 12 students. She makes R1,000 per week for roughly 15 hours of classes — and is no longer worried about exposing her family to the virus.

While professional knowledge workers and creatives have long dominated these platforms, their peak potential lies in attracting a far wider range of creators including low-wage and service workers. There is a future in the hustle economy for teachers, health care workers, and fitness trainers, among other professions. But it's far from clear whether the hustle economy represents a triumph of technological innovation and human creativity or a failure on the part of the traditional economy and the social safety net.

It is not easy sailing though. Workers in the hustle economy remain wholly dependent on the platforms that supposedly empower them. To further paraphrase Karl Marx: Is the platform a tool used by the worker or is the worker a tool used by tech executives? It isn't just that hustle economy platforms take a cut of workers' earnings.

Workers bear enormous up-front costs and risks to produce their work. Should the platform choose to change anything from a payment processing fee to a recommendation algorithm worker have no real power to influence those decisions.

It is still very precarious. Hustle economy founders and investors say they're aware of this precarity, though they generally believe creative people will manage to find a way. Mark predicts an ecosystem of support services will spring up around the hustle economy, much as it did around Airbnb.

Briggle doesn't want to be on Patreon forever. This was never her dream, she said. At one point during the shutdown, her husband asked her what she'd like to do if she started over and she cried because she'd open Soma again. Until that point, then, she's sticking with Patreon, the only option she has. To her surprise, more people subscribed to her videos immediately after the country reopened. 'I have to remind myself it's not always going to be this way. I will get to the other side. We will get back to normal again whatever colour, shape or form it takes.'

Sunday, 25th ...2021
Hello South Africa, welcome joy

Hope can feel like an oscillating journey between light and dark, as slippery as an eel, as dangerous as walking blindfolded on a cliff edge. It can feel like clamouring and clawing at thin air. In a world that is at this moment resurrecting in slow motion, from monumental pain and suffering, the expectation that things will get better is the notion that keeps us moving forward. It directs our humanity and our sense of purpose.

Hope is such an awkward and personal perception. The emotional response we have to keep going, to find solutions, will vary. Knowing though, that we are all a part of an interconnected ecosystem that miraculously gives light, air, water and sustenance, that has, over billions of years, provided us with everything that is fundamentally necessary to living, provides the brightest form of loving reciprocity. Look up, look out and within. It beats there, hope.

Then, one morning in September, the sun rose, piercing through the dark clouds that had previously blocked its shine. This is the day our economy's doors were re-opened for business. It coincided with spring equinox. Surely, a sign the universe has aligned its stars to glow on us. I imagine September 21st undergoes a metamorphosis, transforming from a Spring Day to New Year's Day. The ushering of new beginnings appropriately nicknamed After Domestication (AD).

It is a wonderful day to wake up alive, even better to be alive in promise-filled day. Celebs and regular folks alike have taken to verse to voice their joys in birthday bashes and family reunion gigs. The songs about their resentment of lockdown, the wastefulness of waiting. Songs have created popularity records across the musical landscape, none less so than the tuneful *Jerusalema*.

South Africa gave the world the song, the young Ugandan dancers gave it the zeitgeist igniting the world's imagination. The Jerusalema sounds streamed locally and globally, sung by Presidents and Prime ministers, and the Pope was in on the act too. Young men danced to their heart's delight while the old ululated with their voices creating a festive atmosphere. South Africa was ready for the second return of our Lord.

The sounds of joy are booming everywhere, South African is alive with song and dance. You did not have to ask the good times were rolling. Music everywhere, all day deep into the new curfew free hours. The vibes were great. I danced hard. My favourite streaming on Spotify. The Afro House single *Okokoko*, by Sphectacula & DJ Naves featuring Unathi and *Your love* by Azana. The other by Sun-El featuring Msaki. *Ubom Abumanga*.

> 'Bekukudala ngoko useneminqweno
> Khawude uwele iblorho
> Uze nganeno
> Bekukudala ngoko usenazinjongo
> Sasikhule sonke
> Sphupha emazulwini
> Sgcakameli'ilanga
> Yiza ndikukhumbuze
> Ubom' abumanga....'

Music is harmonious, no wander it creates goodwill and friendliness. Music can overwhelm the mind when we hear it, we lose our bearings too. When we hear the gliss of fingers walk across the neck of a guitar, the rhythm of the drums, the singer's voice begins to call and for a moment our mind is transformed, we must do as we are told to follow the beat.

The magic of music beguiles all human beings, we cannot resist it. Sometimes we do not notice how it catches our soul and makes us stop, makes us forget. The rhythms of the soul bring peaceful feelings, and form friendships among the young and tired wayfarers of life. Yes, music calls out to our deeper instincts and causes us to become motivated to live life fully. Music speaks to a higher dialect in our deeper selves. The music in our depths connects us to our true selves and to others.

Many including myself forgot that we were at the adaptation phase not past the pandemic. Adapting from pandemic to endemic stage means we are learning to live with the virus, knowing it is still active in our midst.

After a tiring day, I retired to my studio in quiet, I reverted to what I like best. Writing. Writing is like thinking on paper, to read the thoughts of another is to essentially converse with the writer. In writing my greatest love, or what brings me joy includes translating emotions, and experiences into a coherent, sharable format, sharing it with you, getting your heart, your reactions, your kind words, your reflections. All of it.

My writing is not the greatest, yet I must improve if I must win the Nobel Prize. It is not always crisp, fresh but you never tire of reading my work, in fact you find my work engaging. I give you a clue to success in so many of my titles. I am so thankful that I could openly share how I have done it. Indeed, the best things in life are not only free but priceless.

If I am alive, I shall be a student. Learning about the self, through healing, acceptance, strangers, elders, research and even going back to start all over again. Learning about other traditions, about Artificial Intelligence, food, anything that sparks my curiosity.

One of the many gifts of experiencing the dark side of waiting, it allows me to experience the light fully. After being single for years, I am in love again. While it is a new relationship, the emotional intimacy brings me into the present moment, and opens my heart in ways I did not know were possible.

Relationships do encourage good behaviours that work for us, which improves our mood, and wellbeing. So, it makes sense that studies show having fewer social ties is associated with health problems. The person I choose to surround myself with has a bigger impact on happiness and total well-being than I initially thought.

Social connections with friends make us a lot happier. Satisfying relationships not only make us happy but they also give us better health and longer life. It is our nature, and we cannot live our lives without social interactions. Friends play a crucial role in our happiness.

Being with close friends, who I can laugh with, admit my sins to and be fully myself without any act. The friends I hold dear when they are in distress because they trust me enough to let go. The friends that show up when life is hard and sit there and listen. I owe my survival during this pandemic to my close friends, and they know who they are. You, my friends, bring me joy.

After all, never have a hand touched love. Never has an eye spotted peace. Never has a nose sniffed dream. Why do I feel like I want to sit down, have coffee with you, and argue over these assertions? To be human is to feel. To have the privilege of our brains lighting up at the enjoyment of a field of tulips in our vision, the scent of sweet roses.

Some men chase women, some women chase money, some of both chase Vodka with a mixer of choice, yet every chase leads to the same pot at the end of the rainbow, happiness. Joy said Aristotle is the meaning and the purpose of life, the whole aim of human existence. For a joyful life, choose to value meaningful work, deeper relationships, and the freedom to fully express yourself and be who you truly are.

Deep yourself in silent meditation. Nature. Quiet Sunday afternoons with a book. Listening to the sound of the rain. Dancing, working out, yoga, hiking. Anything that allows my body to open, to release, to express without the force of the intellect. In peace, I find my fullest joy. Engaging my creativity is always in a team format: solving a challenge, starting a project, and bringing an idea to life. Supporting and encouraging others to act on their passions. Oh, the joy to witness someone step into her power and bring to life the full repertoire of her gifts.

Connecting, especially with people going through hard times. Letting them feel seen by validating their experience. Showing them they too matter makes them feel hopeful again. The faith. The grit. The power they have within. This brings me joy. I share it freely.

Everyone now is always trying to feel better, to overcome the negative mood they were in not so long ago. The goal is just to feel good again. When we feel happy, we are more likely to sacrifice some of the comforts of old, worn-in relationships to achieve longer-term goals of networking with new friends.

I have a habit of randomly surrendering to life's funny ways. Getting on a bus with no destination in mind. Landing in a city with no plans. One time I spent a night with a group of Rasta Commune I did not know, I met them randomly. We went to karaoke, then food, then their studio and recorded with them. I intentionally keep some days with no plans. Making others laugh. Nothing beats putting a smile on someone's face. I love an audience. I make witty jokes and act silly.

One of the lessons that emerged during my wait was to appreciate freedom. Freedom gives me the opportunity to pursue meaningful things. Freedom has led to enhanced expression of creativity and original thought. The freedom to be who I am, over my time and what to do with it. The freedom to invest in something meaningful. Anything. It was Napoleon Hill who said, 'remember that your real wealth can be measured not by what you have, but by what you are.' Real wealth is the abundance of time and freedom giving me the time to make an impact in someone's life and the opportunity to make a change that matters to her.

People succeed, thrive, and enjoy life by getting curious about who they really are and doing what they value most in life. My core values help me align my actions for the rest of my life with what makes me come alive and create a life based on what gives me joy. You too can change your life immeasurably once you realize that time is your most valued resource. Waiting is fun unfolding one moment a time. That is why I am a fan of waiting. Waiting if done well activates my innate my insights.

Post-COVID-19 lockdown
The ultimate question

'Bae, I know I did not address the question you asked me last night. I have thought it through though. As we begin to glimpse a future free of lockdown, knowing everything we now know I have no doubt in my mind we should have killed the coronavirus on its tracks, and it is not difficult to know how. By an act of waiting. A simple act of waiting would have given us answers we desperately needed at the right time. Waiting would have given us the space to think things through, time to perfect experimental drugs and shield those who needed it most. Besides waiting being an expression of faith in God's providence, axiomatically, waiting is self-evident wisdom. One develops a better perspective when one waits long enough for the dust to settle and letting the haze lift. If there's one place in the world where a mutant variation is likely to happen it will be in an area where you have a high infection rate and no lockdown or a vaccine programme. That's us.

The Bible says, 'be patient as you wait because how you wait is the key to your breakthrough,' it further says, 'when you are patient, you lack nothing.' Every adult who has lived long enough can attest to the truthfulness of this statement. While we wait, we suspend both expectation and judgment, prepared to accept any outcome that might present. Because we are not anxious at that exact moment we lack nothing.

Westcott puts it succinctly, 'true life comes from complete self-surrender. In a state of surrender, we become free to enjoy life in the moment. In the bigger scheme of things waiting works to our benefit so that we may enjoy life with the benefits this brings. By surrendering, we step into a higher life over which the power of ego wanting to do this or that has no hold.' Surrender is giving over to higher power and to the deepest emancipation of our vexed self.

This is true on many fronts. Philosophically, scientifically and at the practical level there is evidence for this. Imagine for a second, the world waited and when we emerged from the quarantine adhered strictly to social distancing, face covering and avoidance of any and all mass gatherings in public places including funerals. We would have effectively arrested if not considerably slowing down the development of community transmission clusters.

A successful wait during lockdown would have meant buying scientist time to develop sterilizing immunity vaccines rather than being pushed to produce the less than inadequate effective vaccines thereby gotten out of the pandemic sooner. Indeed we have added eight years to the fight against the pandemic. It is self-evident our salvation rested in the waiting.'

'Bae, I hear you loud. But if it is God's design to use our time on earth to condition us to the strictures of waiting, why is this skill not evident in most, I mean lots of people me included suck at this, right.'

'In our fast-paced world we do not wait, in fact we hate waiting whatever the length or reason. If we must wait, we do so impatiently, often time with great resentment. Because we failed to wait when we were told to do so during the lockdown, the government was forced to revise rules so we could do some activities outside our homes while under quarantine. Shielding was the key focus area. Even so, we cut corners when we followed the mandatory social protocols.

Because of our failure to wait, we enabled conditions where clusters of community transmission became prevalent, widespread, and uncontrollable. Towards the end of the year the virus mutated to highly transmissible variants, coming back stronger the second time, infecting those who should be shielding rendering thereby rendering the hard work of the scientists dump squid.

Wrongly believing that a vaccine is a panacea to the pandemic, we demanded production to be expedited and brought forward ahead of their normal development regime in the process placed scientists in an invidious position where they had to choose between saving those with co-morbidities first or saving everybody at once. A stopgap measure good enough just to keep people from hospitalisation was agreed.

The mess was not resolved by the arrival of the vaccine when the vaccines were available. We could not wait for the medicine to do its job. Considering the weak outcomes yielded by the first generation vaccines, Scientist have had to go back and design second generation vaccines for sterilizing immunity. A short term view is a perfect way to be held hostage by the global pharma companies. Shortcuts, however conceived are never the right way to address a pandemic.

As early as the third month of the pandemic, scientific and general information concerning the virus facing humanity had been made public widely, reaching the masses in the general population. Most knew, for example, we were unable to see the virus as it was too small. We could imagine it. Once the pathogen had entered the human cell, it incubated for a short time before symptoms show up. There was no cure available. What the doctors were doing under the circumstances was hit and miss at best. Reference knowledge from the available drugs was inexact.

We were forewarned that we were vulnerable because we could see the enemy killing us, we have no known cure. And so, the battle cry from the scientific community 'stay the hell away from anything that might expose you to infection and wait in your home until help is found. If you must go to public spaces musk up.' While we showed some restraint in public, privately we told ourselves and anyone willing to hear us, 'to hell with all that we will do what bloody want and fuck to anyone who will to stop us.'

The public health authorities were on the losing side while the virus was winning the battle.

Not only was God present before this crisis and during its reign of terror, but his mercy has been sufficient for us. There is not one day where we were alone in this crisis. Not only does God know what to do, but he also cares. God has never failed his people. We were accompanied by God whose mercy said no. His mercy would not allow the virus ravaging effects to decimate the Afrikan communities because God wants his glory to be on full display.

Although we know what the end of the story will be, we wait for it without knowing when it will come. It may come within our lifetime; it is possible that it may not come during our earthly season. But that is not the reason not to wait.

Our affliction had a purpose and a timeline, even though it already seemed too long. We likely did not know what it was then, someday we will. And we will understand that the purposes for both our affliction and how long we were required to endure it extended far beyond the range of our perception. And then it will make sense. I am thankful for the lockdown. In the end, it was for my benefit. This is God's way to make me wait, so that in my waiting I may see his plan. Clear and full picture.'

Where do we go from here is the question that cannot be answered by governments of the world of science? Only God can answer it for us God's timing is always impeccable his word infallible.

∞∞∞∞∞∞

Postscript

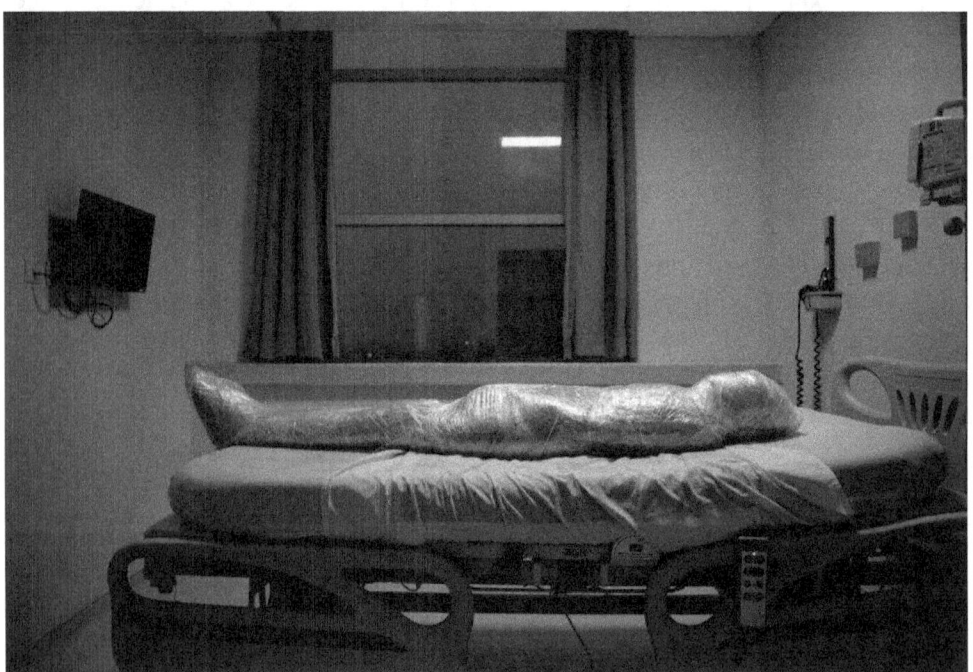

This body on the hospital bed came as a patient now leaves in shrink-wrapped plastic destined for disposal at an unmarked city grave

Source: TIME Magazine December 2020

By same author

Fractured Hope: South Africa reflects upon the future of her children
Let it be known I am God of heaven and the earth
Matthew 6: 33: Seeking the face of our Father
96th Thesis: miracles, money, and strange fires
State Capture: truth eclipses the shadows
A story about waiting
Letters for my Sons
A different time
Ek is 'n Qriqua
Commissioned
Joie de vivre
Sorry earth
Live loud
1632

Endnotes

Accurate information is an indispensable tool for honest writing. The subject of coronavirus is new to most of us, I consulted websites listed below for data I believe reliable. Johns Hopkins and WHO are experts in global public health, infectious disease, and emergency preparedness and have been at the forefront of the international response to COVID-19. Their websites are dependable resources to advance the understanding of the virus and guide a response, improve care, and save lives. Commentaries on the handling of the coronavirus by state actors does not meet the same stringent criteria, however. Readers are advised to exercise caution when interacting with information from these websites.

Hornby Gill. 1965. Miss Austen. Penguin Books.
Howard, B C. 2016. Seasons of Waiting: Walking by faith when dreams are delayed. Crossway
Kendi, Ibram X. 2016. How to be an Antiracist. Penguin.
Luther, Martin. 1664. Luther's Works, Volume 43. Banner of Faith
Snowden, F, M. 1956. Epidemics and Society: From the Black Death to the Present. Harvard Press
Vroegop, M. 2019. Dark clouds, Deep mercy: discovering the grace of lament. Crossway
Vroegop, M. 2020. Weep with Me: How lament opens the door for racial reconciliation. Crossway
www.who.int/public/emergencies/coronavirus
www.coronavirus.jhu.edu/data
www.psomagen.com/the-viral-evolution-of-covid-19
www.sciencemag.org/the-pandemic-appears-to-have-spurred-africa-so-far/08/2020
www.humanparts.medium.com/matt-gough-memoir-of-a-white-brother/06/2020
www.webmd.com/what-you-need-to-know-about-coronavirus/htlm.06/2020
www.webmd.com/disease-has-not-changed-but-scientific-understanding-has evolved/html.07/2020
www.ncbi.nlm.nih.gov/pmc
www.specialprojects.news24.com/south-africa-beyond-covid-19./html.06/2020
www.news24.com/servaas-van-der-berg-poverty-rises-inequality/htlm.06/2020
www.theconversations.com/news-analysis
www. scroll.in/article/i-was-on-the-who-team-that-went-to-wuhan23/02/21
www.theeconomist/measuring-the-poverty-pandemic/07/2020
www.historicalpapers-atom.wits.ac.za/papers-HPRA
www.phylosophy.org. | Issue 96 | Philosophy Now| Waiting.
www.bbc.com/why-vaccinated-people-may-still-be-able-to-spread-covid19/20210203?
www.theeconomist.com/won't-know-much-about-history/07/2020

www.ingramcontent.com/pod-product-compliance
Lightning Source LLC
Chambersburg PA
CBHW060831220526
45466CB00003B/1056